C000193721

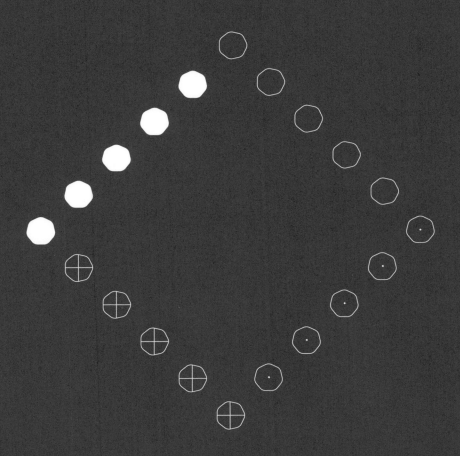

BENTO POWER

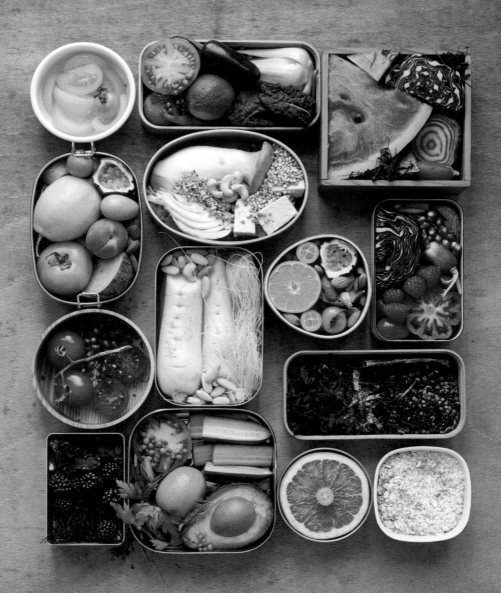

Brilliantly Balanced Lunchbox Recipes

Sara Kiyo Popowa

of

Shiso Delicious

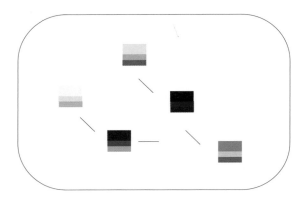

An Hachette UK Company
www.hachette.co.uk

First published in Great Britain in 2018 by
Kyle Books, an imprint of Octopus Publishing Group Limited
Carmelite House
50 Victoria Embankment
London EC4Y 0DZ
www.kylebooks.co.uk

ISBN: 978 0 85783 499 7

Text copyright 2018 © Sara Kiyo Popowa
Design and layout copyright 2018 © Octopus Publishing Group Limited
Photographs copyright 2018 © Sara Kiyo Popowa

Sara Kiyo Popowa is hereby identified as the author of this work in accordance with section 77 of the
Copyright, Designs and Patents Act 1988.

All rights reserved. No part of this work may be reproduced or utilised in any form or by any means,
electronic or mechanical, including photocopying, recording or by any information storage and
retrieval system, without the prior written permission of the publisher.

Photography and Styling: Sara Kiyo Popowa *
Graphic Design: Before Breakfast Design Ltd
Project Editor: Sophie Allen
Production: Nic Jones and Gemma John

* except portraits of Sara: Andy Towers (page 8); Carolina Llamusi-Silbermann (pages 11, 16, 52);
Jenna Foxton (pages 70, 98, 162, 192).

A Cataloguing in Publication record for this title is available from the British Library.

Printed and bound in China.

10 9 8 7 6 5 4

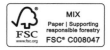

CONTENTS

MY STORY

To tell you about my bento would be impossible without telling you a little bit about myself and the part food has played in my life. There are quite a few things to say, so let's get started!

Sweden

It all began in Sweden in the 1970s. My mum, who was living in Sweden with her Bulgarian dissident parents, fell in love with my dad, a Japanese student of Nordic history. They got married and moved to Japan. My mum found being a non-Japanese woman in Japan challenging, especially as my dad's family household was very traditional. When she was pregnant with me, she decided to return to Sweden – just a few weeks before I was born.

My first years were spent with my grandparents in the countryside of southern Sweden, surrounded by fruit trees, rose bushes and tiny insects, while my mother retrained as a nurse. My granddad was always doing some sort of building project or cooking up big feasts while my grandmother worked as a doctor in the local hospital. Soon, my Swedish stepdad arrived, and soon after, little brothers.

We then relocated to Norrland. Yep, Norrland. It's a sparsely populated region of northern Sweden, full of spruce forests and lakes, with intensely light summers and dark, cold winters. I spent half the year playing in the snow and reading, drawing and making things indoors. The other half was full of bright, long days, mosquitos, endless open nature and foraging for berries with my brothers.

I was one of the rare 'non- Swedish' kids in my school. At this stage, my Japanese heritage and biological father were abstract concepts to me – a far, far away world. As this was long before the internet, I, like everyone else around me, knew very little about Japan – they eat with chopsticks? Geishas come from there, right?

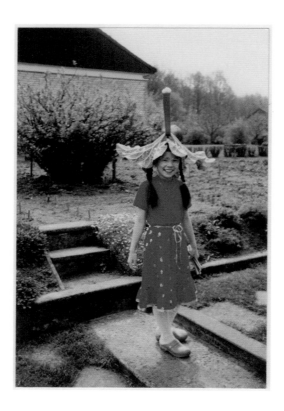

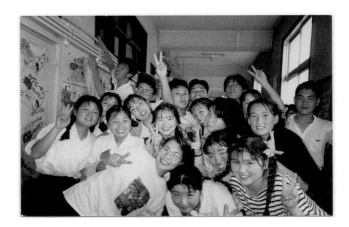

Getting to know Japan

As a 17-year-old, I went to Japan for a year on a student exchange. Student life in Japan was very different to liberal 1980s Sweden. I wore a school uniform and lessons were delivered with no teacher-student dialogue – just be quiet and do as you're told! I felt a rebellious nature bubbling-up in me, something I hadn't felt back home.

At lunchtime, we'd pull our desks together and unpack our bento boxes. Most students would bring one, although there was a cafeteria selling snacks. I got the feeling that if you relied on the cafeteria for lunch, there may be something a little wrong with your family situation. My host family Takaya-san's mother would pack my bento in a cute little box every morning. She'd start with rice: sometimes plain, sometimes seasoned, sometimes shaped into onigiri rice balls. She'd then add the side dishes (o-kazu) – anything from fish, omelette, meat, beans or vegetable dishes (cooked especially to make bento for the family) to ready-bought sides or dinner leftovers. There would always be some Japanese pickles and seaweeds but rarely plain raw vegetables. She'd then pack the bento-box in a bento bag, or tie it into a colourful handkerchief (furoshiki) along with a pair of character-adorned chopsticks in their own little carrying case. My excitement of taking all those cute accessories to school every day was immense!

During this time, I met my Japanese dad for the first time. Looking back, I'm unsure who was more confused by the situation, him or me. Our relationship didn't really take off although, many years later, we have reached some sort of peace. Despite that, I was intrigued by the country responsible for half of my roots: its people, the culture and the possibilities it offered away from quiet Sweden. I now knew I was not going to settle back into my life back home.

My relationship with Japan continued as a university student, first on an exchange with my Stockholm University course and then on a year in Tokyo on a scholarship at Sophia University. The Japanese Ministry of Education would be horrified if they knew I spent most of my year clubbing and attending only one of my classes – Japanese language. On the bright side, I was fully immersing myself in Tokyo life, becoming fluent in the language and making lots of Japanese friends.

My relationship with food

While in Japan (and, incidentally, while trying to create some sort of relationship with my father), my relationship with food/eating started to become unbalanced. As a teen in Norrland I'd been used to eating as much as I wanted and still being the tiniest person in my class. In Japan, I was suddenly taller than many middle-aged men (much to their age-and-gender-hierarchical annoyance) and surrounded by diet-obsessed waifs of girls who seemed to survive on sweets alone. Oh and those snacks were amazing too – all the inventiveness of Japanese food culture blossomed in the (high-quality) junk and convenience food that was available at every step in public, at every hour.

I had already started to have insecurities about my body since moving out of my slim teenage years and as my cheeks chubbed out I began to feel stressed and ashamed eating the amounts I wanted. While at university, I started dieting, which soon turned into a full-blown eating disorder that stayed with me in shifting form for over a decade. Even though I hid it well, it affected every single aspect of my life, whether or not I realised it at the time.

While becoming more aware of food, my body and human nature, I stopped eating meat. I didn't want to feed my body with something that was so similar to myself, that had been killed. I would say I was the only vegetarian I knew in Japan!

When I had finished my scholarship in Japan, I decided to go back to Europe. I settled for London. It was the first place I'd visited where I'd instantly felt 'normal'. It had the big city buzz like Tokyo but I felt there was so much more potential to find whatever I was looking for here – unlike in Japan where I'd have to conform to the strict social norm (literally becoming Japanese) or forever be a 'foreign' oddity.

London proved to be a place you can dream up whatever you like – a few months after arriving, I was hand-crafting my own line of clothes (hand-painted underwear!), which I sold at Portobello and Spitalfields markets, whilst working part-time in a health-food shop. I'd been thrilled to discover that being veggie was pretty normal here, actually there was quite a big 'green scene', which I soon felt at home in. For the next few years, I'd try every type of food, diet and alternative remedy there was, while reading books on Ayurveda and traditional Chinese medicine (and a fair amount of 'crystal healing' too!). I got introduced to the concept of elements (water, earth, fire, air), which defined the way I look at many things. This deep-dive into the healing potential of food was, of course, driven by me wanting to heal my relationship with it – and ultimately the relationship with myself.

Whilst experimenting with food, I became acutely aware of the different effects it had on my body and how different ways of eating (or not eating) triggered different aspects. Lightness, heaviness, stimulation, suppression, flavours, colour – I was longing for a resolve but the path was long and winding. I was cooking A LOT. Despite my struggle, food still meant home and love. In retrospect, love, trust and respect for myself is what I was desperately looking for. It's hard to trust in oneself though, if you don't really know who you are!

Eventually I was ready to go back to studying – and this time something I really wanted to do – art related to the body. I completed a degree in Dance and Visual Art and trained in Butoh, a Japanese post-war performance practice. Immersed in art and performance, something shifted. What had needed an outlet had found it. I stretched everything I knew about being comfortable in front of other people, challenging my audience as much as myself. My secret monsters were allowed to surface and you know what happened to the troll, when it saw daylight? Yep, it exploded (according to Swedish folklore!).

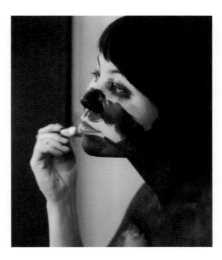

As I was becoming more at home in, and proud of, what my body could do, I also lived with someone who ate three hearty meals a day and never seemed to think much about it (or gain any weight!). Seeing this up close helped too, and gradually, I dared to eat what and when I needed to, to feel energised. I was slowly becoming clearer and more productive. My burning desire to express the strangeness of human nature was fading. As I changed, my friendships and relationships changed too. One day (or very late one night actually!) I met someone who I soon felt I wanted to grow old with. This was Andy, my love and main bento-receiver!

In this new state – simply explained as 'happy' – I moved back to London and spent time nesting while working as a graphic designer (which, somewhere in there with the art and the food had crept in as a bread earner). I missed having my own creative outlet, but I had nothing in particular to say. Until...

Bento Power!

Bento originates from a culture where ritual and presentation plays an important part of daily life, and where a lot of focus and energy goes into producing, cooking, eating and talking about food. A bento is one neatly packed portion of food you take with you to work or school, prepared at home or bought ready-made on your way to work.

When I first met Andy, I was surprised to see him eating out 4–5 days a week, even though he was sporty and enjoyed healthy food. His lunch would either be something beige from his work canteen or a sad chain-store sandwich. How could I rescue him from this de-energising food?

The answer came during our first trip to Japan together. We spent a week on Yakushima, a mountainous island covered in ancient cedar forest where we found a family-run shop making the most incredible, rustic bento which we took with us on our forest hikes. These bento, along with remembering the ones my host family Takaya-san's mum would prepare for my school lunches, made me ask Andy that if I made packed lunch a bit Japanese-ish, in a stylish container, would he take it to work? He said yes! And I did too ;) And so, armed with a few cute purchases, I started making bento as soon as we were back in London.

I love the concept and structure of bento – a box of delicious treasures to look forward to at lunch. What I don't love so much about typical Japanese bento is that it's heavy on meat and deep-fried food and stingy on veggies. Recipes usually involve hard-to-find Japanese ingredients, lots of sugar and too many processed ingredients to make any sense. They are also time-consuming to make! So, how are my bentos different? And why did I start making them?

Shiso Delicious

Here I'll start with a confession: the longest I've ever worked in an office is only about two months! Seeing what my colleagues ate there was a real eye-opener. I realised people were surviving on lifeless food day in and day out – food that might fill a gap temporarily, but that would not sustain anyone long term. It seemed like a ticket to not being able to perform your best and creeping health issues. Plus, the amount of plastic packaging flooding the office bins at lunch hour was enough to have me running for my packed lunch!

I started making my own packed lunch then (and even had my first ideas of writing a book, to help people like my colleagues!), but they were not so much bentos, as clip-lock boxes with combinations of raw vegetables, pulses, nuts and killer dressings that I'd put in my box, give a shake and let it marinate in the fridge overnight (and bring with a packet of oat- or rice cakes).

Shortly after this office stint, I met Andy.

Making bentos has became a daily gift to Andy (and to myself when I make one for me too) and an investment not only in our health but also our bond as a family. Taking some time out to create something that brings a little 'home' into our work days casts a protective, magic veil over our health. All while contributing less to the crazy plastic waste situation that we are in right now! I feel that anyone with a busy, modern life can do with more of this.

So what does Andy say? He has never felt more energetic. He no longer experiences 'that afternoon slump', his skin and eyes are clearer and, from a medical perspective, his cholesterol level, which was high around the time I started making him bentos, reduced to normal in two years. I cannot, of course, promise this will happen to everyone who starts eating healthy homemade lunches, but I can see how it's improved Andy's life and it has mine, too. He's now so used to eating well for lunch he will make his own bento when I don't have time and many of his work-mates have started bringing their own lunches as well. This makes me really happy.

During a second trip to Japan with Andy, this time to visit my father, I fell in love with Instagram. When travel photos stopped being exciting, I started uploading pictures of our meals. I had no idea at the time that there were online communities, or which hashtags to use. I was just excited to create something of my own every day that I could show in a public space with just a few taps of my fingers! It wasn't long until I found myself in a creative, inspiring community of people as deeply into healthy food and visual beauty as myself. I had found a new home, and a new training area, stage and audience, too.

When we were in Japan I bought a packet of shiso seeds to take home to London. While uploading my food snaps to more and more followers I was growing shiso like mad in our little London garden. Shiso is a herb with big, pretty fringed leaves, related to both mint and basil, uniquely tasting of 'Japan'. You may know it as a garnish for sashimi – next time try eating it! To me it had always been one of those ingredients I loved but could never find over here, so to be growing my own – with seeds from my father's distant land – was an incredible feeling. When I needed a new name for my Instagram account and website, Shiso just had to be in there – Shiso Delicious was born!

Bento Babies

It's time for bento to fly into the world! To bounce into your lunch, breakfast or even dinners, sneakily getting past dull ingredients and complicated methods and filling you with bento power! I'm excited to share the ideas, methods and tricks I've developed over the past years, that enable me to bento every day. I am super grateful for each and every one of you who read, look at and take something from my quest for better food, less waste and more beauty and love for you, me and our earth. Without your support my mission would never be.
So fly, bento, fly!

Sara x

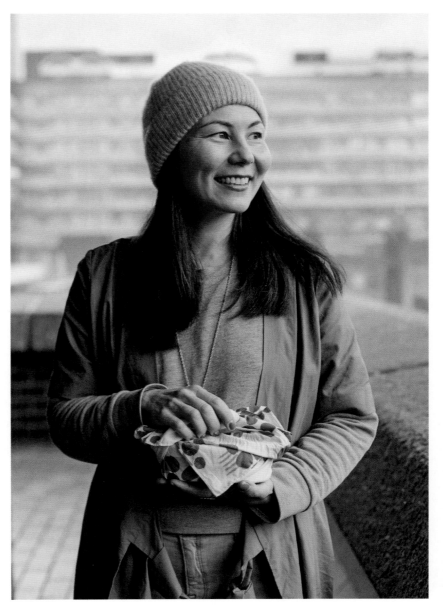

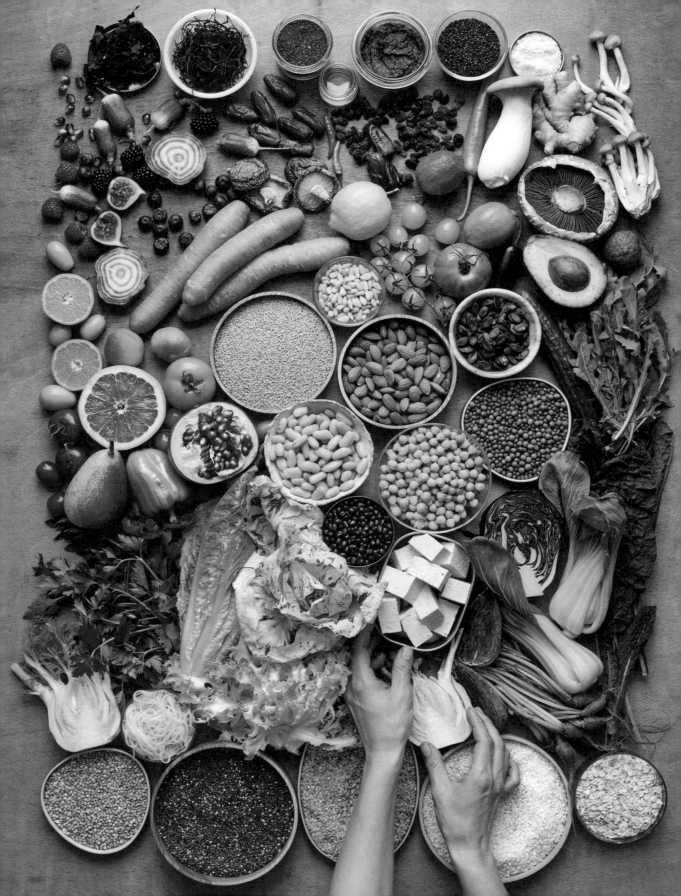

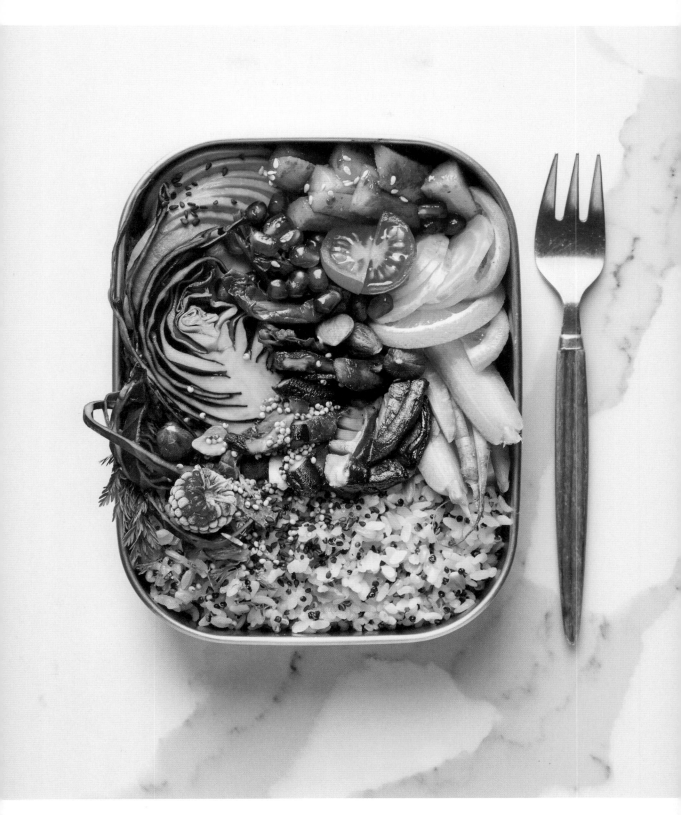

What is a Bento?

With bringing your own lunch and meal-prep becoming so popular you could wonder whether just putting your food in a bento box makes it a bento. Yes and no! To me, the bento format is flexible to include any food you like, but looking at its Japanese origin, there are a few things that make a bento what it is.

The food

A bento is based on the Japanese everyday meal. That is, rice bowl in one hand, eating it chopstickful by chopstickful together with bites of many small dishes, served in many small bowls. Each dish is made to taste, look and feel different, while still complementing each other, and the rice. The very simplest example is one bowl each of rice, miso soup, grilled fish and pickles to eat with the rice. Even though there are a few elements, each can be made very simply (and often appreciating the natural form and flavour of each main ingredient). But yes, as you may have guessed – there's a lot of washing up to do!

A bento is the boxed-up version of this way of eating. Rice, yes, because it is the Japanese (and Asian) backbone, and many small dishes, yes, because that is how the rice is made interesting to eat. Food history tells us that while my ancestors were hard at work harvesting crops from the land, grains were the overwhelming bulk of their diet. Other dishes would have been accents, treats of whatever was available at the time.

The way of packing

So, we have rice, we have small dishes. Now is it a bento? Almost there – we need to pack it in a box (more about the box itself soon), another thing that makes it a bento! In Japan, visual presentation is very important, in food and in culture, in general. As with many other activities, packing bento is rooted in practicality and blossoms in attraction.

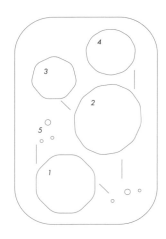

If you've seen Japanese-made bento box containers in real life, they may have seemed small, and this is not just to do with portion size. The food is packed snug, like an edible puzzle, a game of colourful tetris, and the size of your box reflects this. You want to maintain that feeling of sitting down, with all your little dishes and rice, in your bento meal too. The components are neatly grouped, using separators if needed (I like using bits of salad leaves) so that when opening up your bento at lunchtime, it looks the same as when it was packed at home.

Packing like this also means less space for air in your box, so the food stays fresh for longer. This is important as bento is made fresh each morning, and once taken to work or school, it is *not* put in the fridge, but kept and eaten at room temperature. Typical bento dishes are designed with this in mind though, so no need to worry about food safety!

The accessories and ritual around it

The clever little bento is doing a day's work, just like you.
Once bento is filled with nourishing food, it gets wrapped in a pretty cloth, or a dedicated
bag, which makes it present-like as well as hygienic.
Unwrapping at lunchtime, there's a double sense of present. 'Now my lunch starts and I will
take the time to enjoy it.'
While eating, you can use your bento-wrap as a mini-tablecloth.
Packing everything up once you've finished eating is an important part of the ritual.
Neatly pack it up as it came; cutlery, bento box, bento-wrap.
Ready for the journey home!
At home, bento will have a shower and a rest, before being filled up for another day.

PACKING A BENTO BOX

My bento has less small dishes, more greens and often more raw components than typical Japanese bento, so the way I pack it is adjusted to this.

1. Start with rice/grains in one end of the box (or, if using a double-decker box, you could fill one box with rice and the other with the fillings). Pack the grains all the way to the top edge of the box, so they don't move around in transit. I like to make a small slope at the end of the rice, and add juicy fillings on top which flavours the rice.
You can, especially if you use a narrower, deeper box, or a round box, make a bed of rice and place your fillings on top.

2. Here is my Shiso-trick for getting leafy greens in, I make a comfy, pretty bed for the rest of the fillings from salad greens. Before placing them in your box, you can shred the lower half of the salad leaves (the less visual part) and use that as your bed, and save the pretty top parts to frame your creation, or use as separators between fillings.

3–4. Next, put proteins in, and fruit/veg which are bulky and should fill up the space. If there's still space to fill, use raw fruit and veg cut simply to complete your puzzle.

5. Finish with sprinkles/boosts. Here's a chance to balance your bento – if there's not already a lot of protein or fat in your bento, add a few generous spoonfuls of seasoned nuts and seeds or gomashio (sesame salt).
If the bento is already looking very filling, add something for colour and freshness, like tangy pomegranate seeds or herbs. If the bento is lacking in flavour or nutrients, add some of the liquid seasoning potions or furikake – seasoning and nutrient sprinkles.

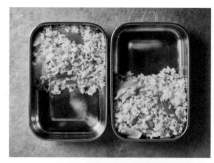

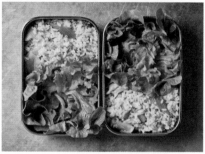

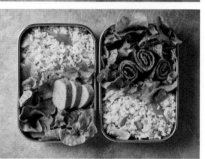

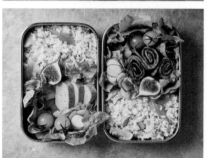

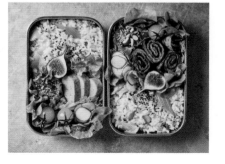

1
2
3
4
5

Furoshiki – bento wrap

Being introduced to bento by my host-mum while in Japan as a teen, I was also introduced to wrapping and transporting my bento in a dedicated cloth (furoshiki) or a soft fabric bag.

Furoshiki is a square, thin, strong cloth (between 40–60cm square), often in a beautiful colour, which goes back to the days when there were no plastic carrier bags and you needed something to carry your shopping in. Remember what I said about the aesthetics of Japan being strongly rooted in practicality! The zero-waste movement (creating a minimum of waste in your personal life) has picked furoshiki up as a reusable, plastic-free way to carry and organise belongings – just as originally intended.

This wrap/bag is just as essential as the box itself, to stop your bento going naked into your work bag! A large fabric napkin (like the linen one in the images, and overleaf), or a fabric tote bag (pictured overleaf) will do just fine, just keep it exclusively for your bento box and wash it regularly.

Bento Box

Your bento box doesn't have to be fancy at all – I started with a simple clip-lock container – but eventually you may want to upgrade to a 'real' bento box. Whatever you use, your box needs to be:

- The right size to hold the portion you want. It's important that the contents fit snugly as explained on page 14.
- Easy enough to transport, standing up, inside your work bag (to stop your edible jigsaw getting messed up). A double-decker (two-tier) box can be great for this as they stack high and narrow.
- Good looking. Part of the fun of a bento is that it should make you happy to look at as well as eat!
- Optional: Leak-proof. You'd be surprised how many bento boxes made for the Japanese market are not, as typical bento food is made not to be wet.

Find your own bento box size by filling an eating bowl you know holds a good portion for you with water, then tip the water into a measuring jug. Good bento boxes and storage containers should state their volume.

Bento boxes come in stainless steel, plastic, or wood, either as single boxes or as double-deckers. Mostly, food for bento is designed not to be too wet, so you can get away with a non-leak-proof box depending on the food you pack (or pack wet foods like dressings in a separate container). In this book, I state when a particular recipe needs to be packed in a leak-proof box.

Cutlery

Packing your own cutlery means you will be prepared whatever happens, and never have to rely on single-use ones! I prefer cutlery made from wood or coconut husk, as they're light and can be packed as they are as they won't scratch the box or accidentally stab something in your work bag.

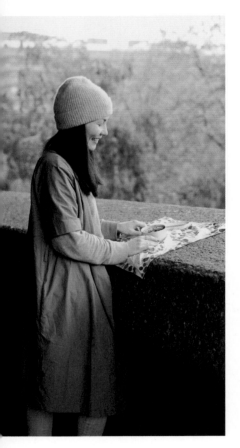

Unwrapping at lunchtime, there's a double sense of present. 'Now my lunch starts and I will take the time to enjoy it.'

WRAPPING A BENTO BOX IN A FUROSHIKI

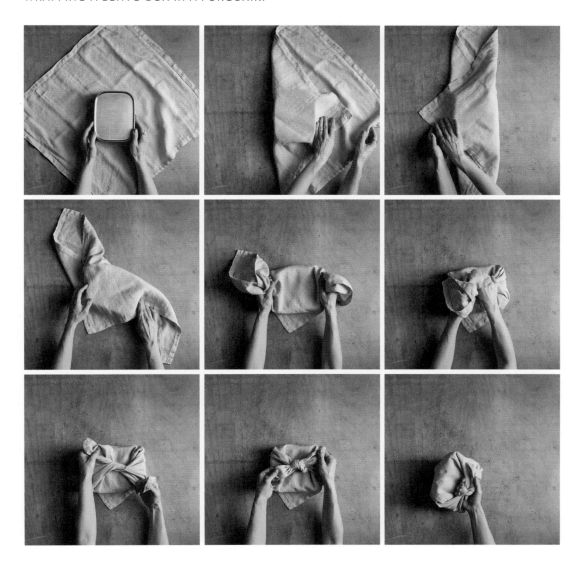

Tools to make Bento

Apart from a bento box and bento carrying wrap/bag I use a few simple, multi-use, good-quality tools. See Resources on page 191 for the brands I use, and where to find them.

1. A sharp knife and a good, clean cutting board

Cutting veggies into bite-sized, good-looking chunks is so much more fun, and faster and easier with a good knife (pictured). If you don't already have a decent one, it doesn't have to cost that much and will really level up your cooking for years to come. I prefer bamboo cutting boards (pictured), and I keep them all, apart from one, free from onion or garlic. This means that every cut veggie keeps their own flavour.

2. Glass jars, storage containers and materials

I use non-reactive materials like glass, enamel and stainless steel both to prepare and store bento dishes. You can put ingredients straight into a glass jar (pictured), shake to combine, pack a portion for your bento then store leftovers in the fridge. I use repurposed, tiny glass jars and small custom bento containers (pictured) for dressings and snacks.

Sturdy plastic bags, like ziplock freezer bags, are practical for quick-pickling, but of course they add more plastic to our seas, so I wash and reuse my bags (just like my grandmother).

I use baking paper both to prepare and store food, and to make little envelopes to pack nuts and sweets into a bento (page 116).

Wax wraps are beeswax-infused natural cloths that I use as a sustainable alternative to clingfilm. Maybe our grandmothers used something similar! They last for ages and are easy to find online (page 191). They are great to wrap onigiri, onigirazu and sandwiches in, too.

3. Rice cooker

This may be the one tool that has enabled Andy and I to keep making daily bentos over the past years. To anyone wanting to eat more rice (other grains can be cooked in a rice cooker, too) they remove a huge chunk of time and concern. Your rice never burns and there's no waiting around. Just load washed rice and water, turn on (or turn the timer on) and come back to freshly cooked rice when it suits you (always perfectly cooked if you follow the rice/water ratio on page 29). Pictured is my ancient but still impeccable little rice cooker. I recommend getting the smallest cooker you can, even if you are a family. It will take up less space in your kitchen and even my tiny '1–2 person' one cooks enough for 4–5 people in one go.

4. A mandolin and/or julienne slicer

These are used a lot in East Asian cuisine and will make preparing raw vegetables a lot faster and more efficient. More fun too! I really recommend getting one, again this is another tool that will really up your bento/cooking game! If you buy just one, buy a mandolin (pictured) and choose a compact design with the least possible parts. My favourite julienne slicer is a simple heldheld Thai one (pictured on page 191).

5. Box or microplane grater

Essential for finely grating ginger, which is used a lot in my recipes (pictured).

6. Not 100% essential, but will make your life a lot easier:
Salad spinner – I use my sturdy 'herb'-spinner both for leaves and to instant-dry noodles.
Egg slicer – speeds up adding overnight eggs to your bento. (page 51).
Handheld julienne slicer – I use a simple Thai papaya salad slicer to make courgetti, so much easier to use and clean than any multi-part 'spiralisers'.
Japanese vegetable brush 'Tawashi' type – natural fibre bristle, clever simple shape, the best!

TIP:
To wash and re-use your plastic bags, fill the bag with a little hot water and a drop of washing-up liquid, trap the air inside and give it a really good shake. Rinse out and hang upside down to dry – I stick mine wet to my kitchen cupboard doors where they will stay until completely dry.

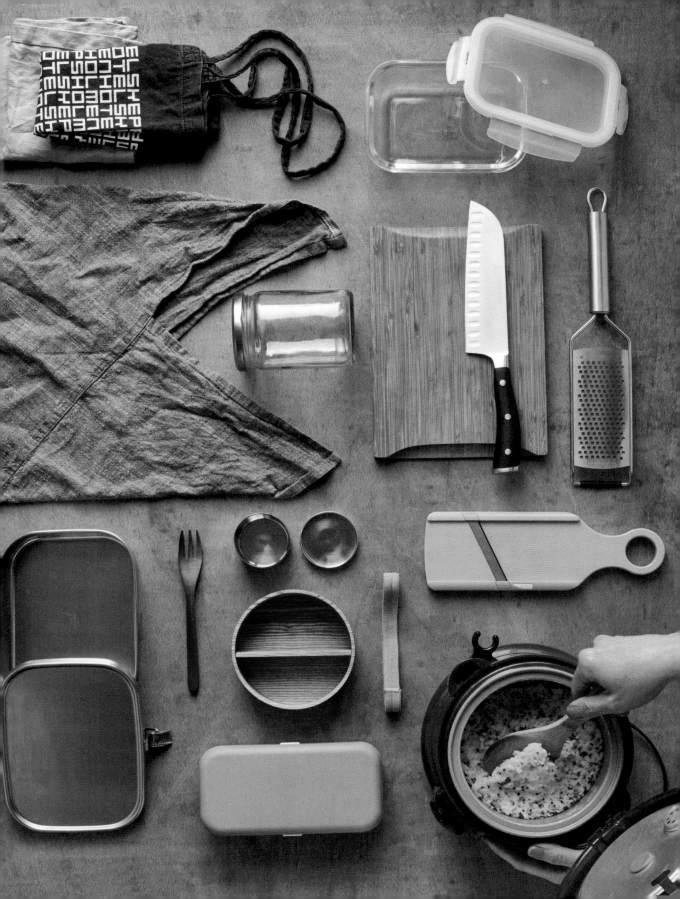

SUSTAINABLE

Having experimented with all kinds of ways of eating, and gone through challenges around it when younger, what is my food like today? What is essential? Apart from being delicious, it's simply 'sustainable'. And this is on every level:

Is it sustainable in how it makes me feel ?

I worked hard to find a balance and now that I have it, I value it so much and I'm not going to lose it! Can I eat like this day in day out and feel 'good'? Can I have clear, even energy and mind (well, most of the time!), feel satisfied, not have crazy mood/energy swings or gain unnecessary weight? By the way, 'having balance' to me includes accepting *not* being perfect.

Is it sustainable to make 365 days a year, for years to come?

Many of us have been there – trying to eat in a way which will never work long-term because it's either too complicated, too expensive, too time-consuming, too alienating, or all of these! Included in this, is understanding that both my body and situation will always keep changing and that I need to stay alert and adjust as I go.

Is it sustainable to my environmental awareness?

Nothing is black and white here. Maybe it's less about 'feeling responsible' for me and more about just *feeling* the general state of our earth and of us here on (with!) it. Feeling this makes me want to do what I can to counteract what's destructive, in any way, big and small.

One of my ways is to work towards the future I would like to see. Another is to reduce that personal waste-mountain I, and everyone else, builds over a lifetime. All whilst saving money so I can choose better-quality food!

Reduce, select, bring and make your own

Only around 10% of everything which is recyclable actually ever gets recycled (globally). Bringing our own food (Bento Power!) and our own reusable containers for drinks is a given. I can't avoid plastic packaging completely but I weigh a few things up when I choose it:

What's its 'volume-timespan' ratio? Is there a lot of plastic for something that will be consumed in one go? (A film-covered tray of ready-made falafels.) Or is it something quite economically packed, that I will get many meals out of? (A bag of dried chickpeas.)

Is there a glass- or metal- packed version of that food? (Then I'll have that please!)

Can I make it myself with ingredients bought in bulk?

Do I *really* need it?

Buying in bulk

This works for me. Even when I've had tiny, shared kitchens, keeping some of my dry staples in bulk has made it easier to eat well. Now I get most of my dried goods in large packets from an online, family-owned whole-food retailer. I find that organic ingredients bought in bulk often works out roughly the same price as for the same non-organic ingredients, in regular volumes in a supermarket.

Basing my diet on plants

I believe we can't continue to 'produce' animals for food at the scale we do now. It is not only extremely taxing on our earth and resources, but causes mass-suffering of other beings.

Support with your spend (and enjoy weaving your community!)

As much as possible I buy organically and small-scale grown, fairtrade and ethically made. I love supporting my fellow local businesses, entrepreneurs, artisans, crafts people, designers and artists with the money I spend. Yeh!

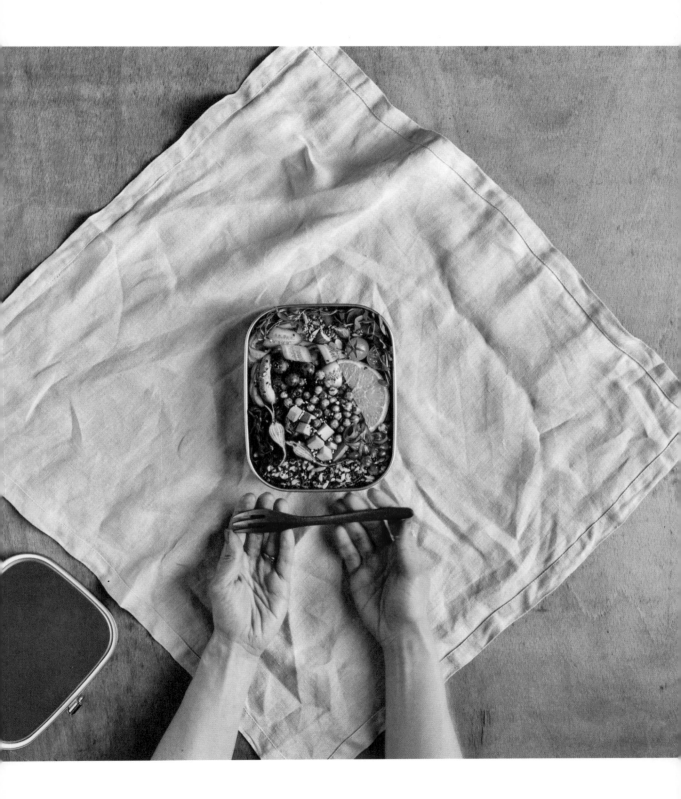

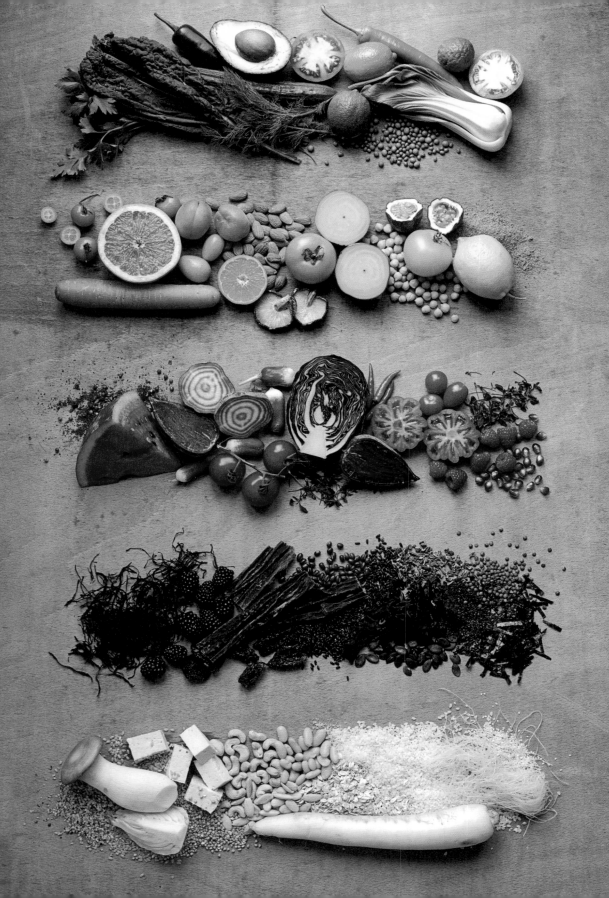

The 5 colours of Shiso Delicious' bento

When I showed my Japanese father the very first image of my Instagram feed – a bento for Andy (which is still up in all its non-photogenic glory), I could tell he was not blown away. After a few moments he said, 'I would want something red in there.'

I immediately felt a little defensive. Sure, I'd put zero styling in and snapped it under the kitchen light. Maybe that was the problem. Red? His comment prompted me to find out about the 5 colours and 5 qualities of Japanese food. And the more I looked, the more I saw them in almost every Japanese meal, even in food packaging design.

A typical Japanese meal should include 5 colours: white, black, red, yellow and green. Looks like Japan had the idea of 'eating the rainbow' for a while already! So in hindsight, the bento my father looked at would have been fine if I'd put a single cherry tomato in there...

Day
Purity
Clear
Space
Calm
Expansion

WHITE / Light Grey / Light Beige
Rice, noodles, white cabbage, cashews, tofu, white beans, egg white, cut radish, cauliflower, white potatoes, white (hulled) sesame seeds, white chicory, cut courgette, cut pear and apple, white currants, coconut, blanched almonds, oats, sunflower seeds, white edible flowers, pine nuts, fennel bulb

Night
Focus
Contrast
Depth
Definition
Earth

BLACK / Dark Brown / Dark Purple
Nori, seaweed, black sesame seeds, soy sauce, black rice, aduki beans, puy lentils, black beans, cacao nibs, purple kale, mushrooms, purple plums, blackcurrants, black pepper, black salt, red shiso, kalamata olives, capers, blueberries, blackberries

Leaf
Growth
Life
Balance
Harmony
Structure

GREEN
Kale, lettuce, avocado, broccoli, fresh herbs, cucumber, green beans, spring greens, pak choi, mizuna, aonori seaweed, pistachios, green peppers, spring onions, chives, fresh green chillies, celery, courgette, peas, kiwi, green shiso, green gomashio, rocket, pumpkin seeds, lime, celery, mung beans, matcha

Blood
Heat
Speed
Movement
Pulse
Fertility

RED / Pink / Purple
Pomegranate seeds, red pepper, tomatoes, gochugaru (Korean pepper), chilli flakes, fresh chillies, red berries, red gomashio, watermelon, radish, beetroot, red cabbage, raddicchio, pink grapefruit, figs, pink pepper, dried goji berries, red pink and purple edible flowers, blood orange, chioggia (candy stripe) beetroot

Sun
Warmth
Happiness
Family
Together
Inclusive

YELLOW / Orange / Light Brown
Tamago, almonds, carrot, sweet potato, squash, banana, citrus fruit, cut nectarines, yellow beets, chickpeas, whole (unhulled) sesame seeds, corn, yellow and orange tomatoes, roasted nuts and seeds, persimmon, yellow plum, yellow pepper, yellow edible flowers, walnuts, conference pear, mango

The 5 elements of Shiso Delicious' bento

Apart from having 5 colours, a complete, traditional Japanese meal should also include 5 flavours (salty, sweet, acidic, bitter and umami/spicy) and 5 different ways of food preparation (raw, steamed, boiled, grilled and fried). This may seem like a lot to keep in mind (and cook), but it's actually quite straightforward!

I see the 5 food preparations as elemental qualities, rather than strict ways of cooking:

Raw (where I include quick-pickled) = cooling, refreshing, cleansing qualities.

Steamed (where I include quick-blanched) = moistening, watery, expanding qualities.

Boiled = stabilising, neutral, bulking qualities.

Grilled (where I include dry-toasted) = drying, smoky, concentrated qualities.

Fried (where I include oven-roasted) = warming, satiating, rich qualities.

I feel that we need a combination of all these qualities and colours in a balanced diet (and life in general) to feel satisfied and nourished.

If you think your bento misses something, or is 'too much', check whether you can add a missing element to balance it. A bento with mainly steamed and boiled ingredients will feel more balanced with a good handful of toasted seeds. A fried- and roasted-heavy bento will be lifted by refreshing raw fruits.

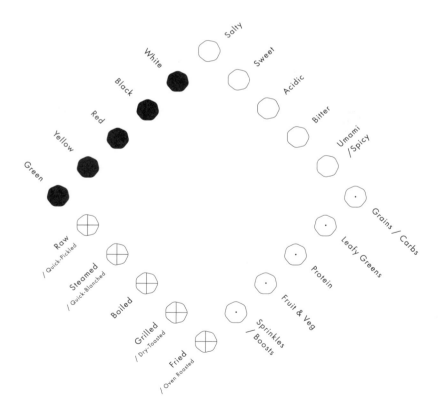

In addition to the traditional qualities, I use the 5 elements below to make my bento, or any of my meals, complete. In a bento where dishes are arranged quite separately, it is useful to think of each dish/filling/component being one of these elements.

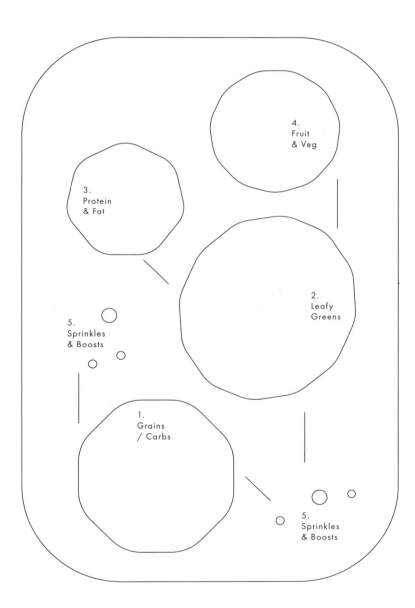

1. Grains / Carbs

Body, endurance and bulk in your bento

Rice, quinoa, noodles, starchy root vegetables

2. Leafy Greens

Cleansing, bitter and balance in your bento

Everything that is leaf, stalk or flower buds on a plant: lettuce, cabbage, spinach, kale, broccoli, oriental greens, spring greens, asparagus, fennel, cauliflower

3. Protein & Fat

Power, stamina and satiation in your bento

Nuts and seeds, pulses, organic egg, tofu, avocado, cold-pressed oils

4. Fruit & Veg

Colour, sweetness and vibrancy in your bento

Fruit: citrus fruit, kiwi, pear, fig, watermelon, banana, plums

Everything that is fruit on a plant: cucumber, pepper, courgette, green beans, tomato

I also include sweet root vegetables here: carrot, beetroot, parsnip, sweet potato, squash

5. Sprinkles & Boosts

Concentrated nutrients and flavour boosts in your bento

Toasted (and seasoned) nuts and seeds, gomashio, furikake, seaweeds, chillies, seasoning sauces and oils, fresh herbs and berries, citrus peel, pomegranate, dried berries, preserved vegetables like olives

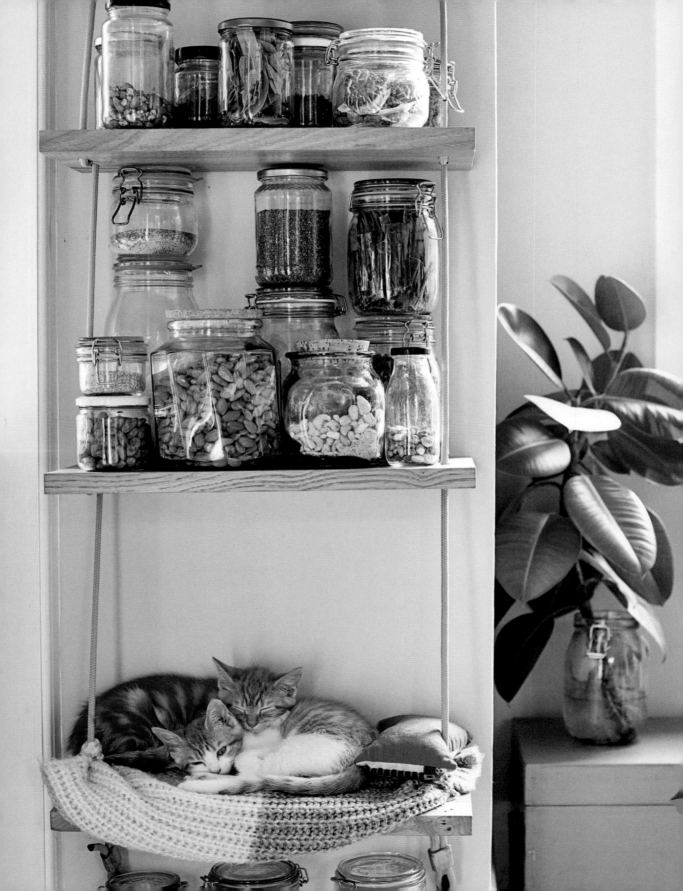

BASE RECIPES

Power up your cupboard and put on a batch of rice! Here I share the secret behind perfectly cooked Japanese rice and how to boost it with other grains and ingredients. All my favourite nutrient-rich seasoning sprinkles are also here, and with a couple of those and a pot of grains you are half-way to making your bento already.

The different rice and sprinkle recipes are interchangeable when used in the 15-minute Bento and Everyday Bento chapters.

Japanese White Rice

This is where it all starts! A child learning how to cook from its parents will first be given the task to wash rice. Cooked right, Japanese white rice has plump, moist grains that are slightly sticky but never mushy – the perfect base for the different flavours and colours of your bento. Once you've mastered cooking rice the Japanese way, you may discover that having it for lunch all year round may be a pretty good idea. There are a few rules and tricks to get that perfect rice, explained here.

When I refer to Japanese white rice, I mean what is sold as 'Sushi Rice', round-grain polished Japonica rice. For more in-depth information about different types of rice, see the section on (Un)usual Ingredients explained on page 182.

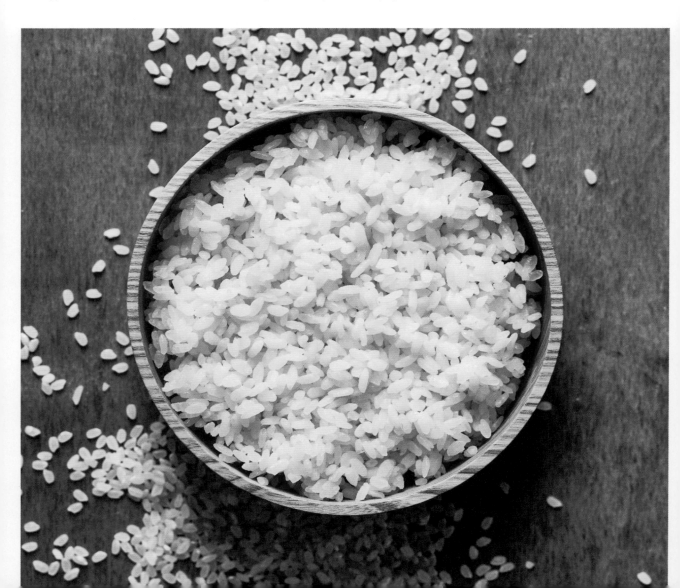

Rule No. 1
Wash your rice in cold water three times

Put the rice in the pan you will cook it in, and make a little bath for it by covering it in a few centimetres of cold water. Then, use your fingers to swirl and 'massage' the grains until the water is very white and cloudy. Pour away this water, using your hand to stop the rice coming out of the pot, breathe, and repeat twice. Washed, Japanese rice won't get mushy when cooked.

Rule No. 2
Use the right amount of water for cooking

Using the right water/rice ratio, all the water will be absorbed by the end of cooking and the rice is neither too mushy or too dry.

All rice recipes in this book have measured amounts of water for cooking, but there's a grandmas' trick if you want to avoid looking at recipes: after washing, level the rice flat (done by adding a little water), then use your index finger as a measuring stick – push it straight into the rice from the top until it touches the bottom of the pan. Note the level the rice comes up to on your finger. You need that same level of water *on top* of the rice. This works perfectly every time, regardless of the amount of rice you're cooking, or the size of your pot. For brown rice, add a few splashes of extra water.

If you have time, soak the rice (once it has been washed) in the measured water for at least 20 minutes, then cook. It really improves the texture!

Rule No. 3
Don't cook with salt

I'm not sure I've ever had a good explanation as to why salt is not added to rice when cooking, but I think it presents a more flexible end result.

The cooked rice is a blank canvas: you can enjoy its purity as it is with the often quite salty Japanese flavours, or fold through, or scatter over seasonings.

Rule No. 4
Don't stir while cooking

Leave the grains to do their thing and get acquainted with their neighbours, without disturbing them.

Rule No. 5
Wait for as long as you can before storing it in the fridge

This may sound against everything you've ever been told. However, cooked, refrigerated Japanese rice gets 'oishikunai' – not delicious – as my host mother would say. I don't live in a hot climate, so for me it works to cook rice in the evening, let it cool overnight, pack a bento in the morning and use leftovers throughout the day or at dinner time. Then I put any leftovers in the fridge and use them either heated up (in a steaming basket, lined with baking paper to stop the grains falling through), fried, or if using as is, revitalised by rubbing some kind of seasoning into it.

Scares about storing and reheating rice are rare in Japan where I often saw cooked rice left at room temperature and never heard of anyone getting sick. It seems those scares originate from the 1970s (!) when restaurant hygiene-control was less regulated here.

A certain spore can be (but is not always) present in rice, which survives cooking and may develop into a bacteria that can cause stomach upset. Every culture with rice as their staple washes the rice before cooking and, personally, I think this may reduce these types of risk. Rice's life is also made longer if you use clean equipment and hands, keep it covered at all times and if you mix the cooked rice with a little vinegar (and salt).

Makes 2–3 portions.
Fridge life: up to 4 days.

Cook Japanese White Rice

I like cooking my rice with a piece of kombu seaweed stuck into it. It's not the classic way, but I like the subtle umami and mineral boost it brings.

220g white Japanese rice
5cm piece of kombu seaweed, optional
350ml water, to cook

Wash the grains with cold water directly in your cooking pot, trying to rub off as much of the cloudy starch as possible with your fingers. Discard the water (by tilting your pot and stopping the grains from falling out with your hand) and repeat twice.

Drain completely, push the kombu into the rice, if using, and add the measured water for cooking (either by using the basic measurements given above, or the finger-measuring hack, Rule No 2). Cover with a lid and bring to the boil, then simmer over a low heat for 15 minutes.

Remove from the heat and, without removing the lid, leave to rest for 5 minutes. If you used kombu, pick it out and mince finely, then gently fold it back into the rice, without crushing the grains too much. Let it cool slightly before packing in your bento and/or a storage container. You can also pack the rice warm in your bento and let it cool off slightly before adding other fillings or closing the lid.

To cook in a rice cooker:

Wash it as above, directly in the (detachable) pot of the rice cooker, add kombu, if using, then cook as per the manufacturer's instructions for standard white rice.

Brown Short-grain Rice

Brown rice is more time-consuming to cook than white, but with that comes a slower release of energy, more complete nutrients and fibre, and a nutty, filling taste – worth the extra time! Brown short-grain is the one most similar in shape and texture to white Japanese rice, and is the one I use throughout this book.

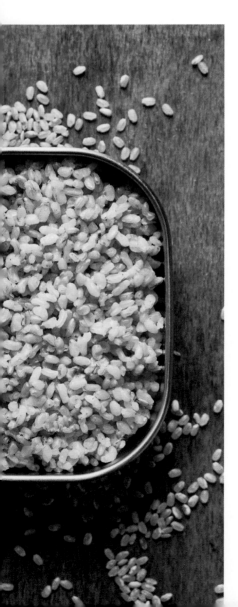

Makes 2–3 portions.
Fridge life: up to 4 days.

Slow-cook Brown Rice

If you have the foresight and time to soak your rice properly, this method makes the tastiest and most nutritious brown rice. A long soak gives certain nutrients that are locked in the dried grain time to release.

220g brown short-grain rice
300ml water, to cook

Wash the rice with cold water once, directly in the cooking pot. Discard the water then add any amount of fresh water to cover (and for the grains to expand a little) and leave to soak overnight or for a minimum of 4 hours.
   Drain, add the measured water for cooking, cover and bring to the boil, then simmer over a low heat for 20 minutes. Remove from the heat and, keeping the lid on, leave it to stand for 10 minutes before using.

Makes 2–3 portions.
Fridge life: up to 4 days.

Quick-cook Brown Rice

Let's face it, there's not always time or foresight to slow-soak brown rice! I started using hot water to speed things up and it works really well.

220g brown short-grain rice
350ml boiling water, to cook

There's no need to wash the rice. Pour plenty of boiling water (any amount) over the rice directly in the cooking pot, cover and leave to soak for 20 minutes.
   Drain off the soaking water, add the measured boiling water for cooking, replace the lid and bring to the boil, then simmer over a low heat for 25 minutes. Remove from the heat and, without removing the lid, leave to rest for 10 minutes before using.

To cook in a rice cooker:

Soak the rice in boiling water as above, drain off the soaking water, add the measured boiling water for cooking, then cook as per the manufacturer's instructions for standard white rice (which is faster than the brown setting) and leave to rest a minimum of 10 minutes before using.

Quinoa

The other week I had a good old friend visiting and we cooked a quinoa recipe from the book. She said she had never toasted quinoa before cooking, or cooked it so that all the water gets absorbed. After hearing this, I thought I'd include how I cook it here. Toasting replaces quinoa's slightly soapy nature with a lovely touch of smoke and dryness and, just like rice, using the right water/grain ratio means you don't have to throw any nutrient-infused cooking water out at the end. Quinoa doubles up as both carbs and proteins, and can be used instead of rice in any recipe in this book.

Makes 2–3 portions.
Fridge life: up to 5 days.

Cook Quinoa

220g quinoa (any colour, or mixed)
400ml water, to cook

Wash the quinoa with cold water once, drain completely and then toast it wet over a high heat in the pot you will cook it in, stirring more frequently as the grains become drier. After 3–5 minutes it will look dry, a little browned and pop a lot. It's fine if it burns slightly as it adds to the flavour.

Add the measured water for cooking, cover with a lid and bring to the boil, then simmer over a low heat until all the water is absorbed and there is no visible white centre in each grain, 15–20 minutes.

Remove from the heat. To cool faster, 'open up' the grains with a very brief stir, then let it steam, uncovered, for 5–10 minutes until it's cool enough to pack in your bento. Let it cool completely before storing in the fridge.

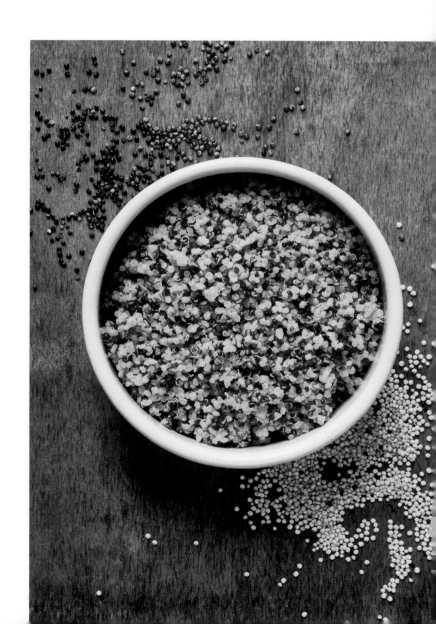

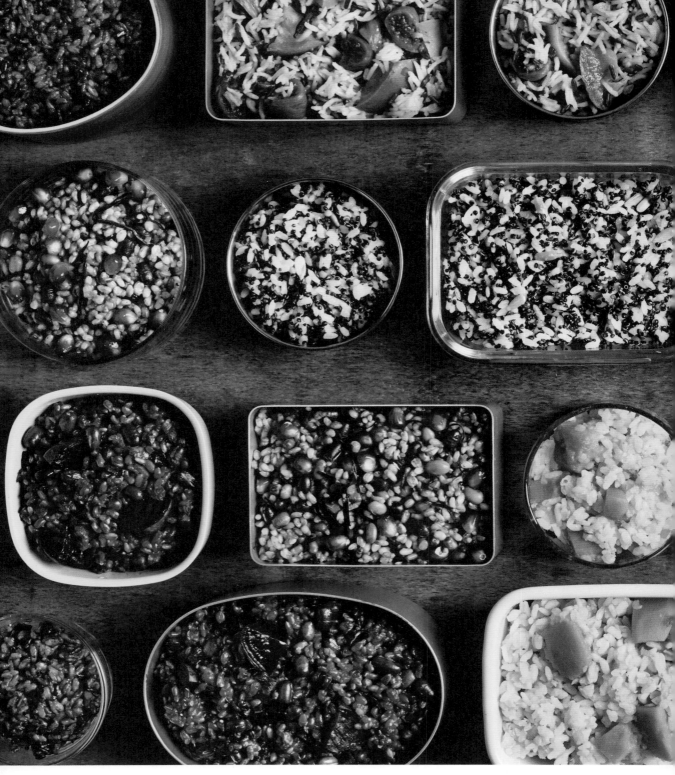

Mixed-grain Rice and One-pot Rice

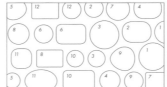

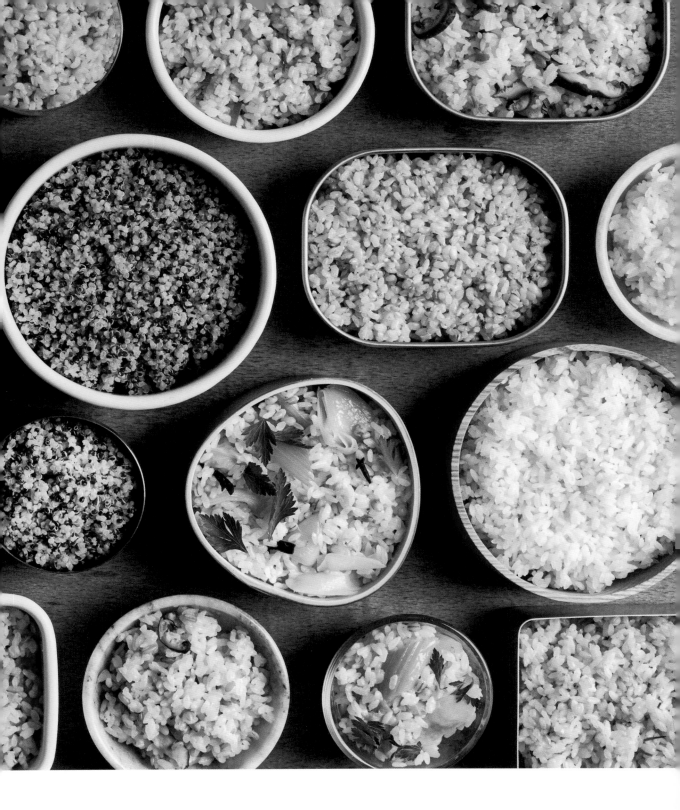

Mixed-grain Rice

White Japanese rice is quicker to cook than brown (and tasty!), but I'm aware it lacks nutrients, especially if eaten regularly. So 'zakkoku-mai', multi-grain rice has become standard in our house. Throwing a few handfuls of whole grains in with your white rice takes just a few moments, and you get more flavour, texture, nutrients and fibre in the same cooking time as white alone. My Shiso twist is using a larger amount of multi-grains than typical recipes, and using ingredients that are easy to source here in the UK.

In my bento recipes I usually suggest a specific mixed-grain or one-pot rice (overleaf) to use, but you can use any.

See page 29 for more detail on how to wash your rice, and how to cool it faster (once cooked), directly in your bento box.

TIP:
To use a rice cooker (for all mixed-grain rice apart from Multi-multi Rice): wash the grains directly in the (detachable) pot of the rice cooker, add extras, then cook as per the manufacturer's instructions for standard white rice.

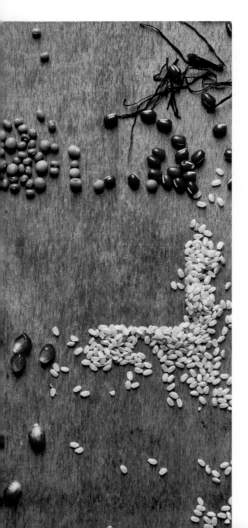

Grainy Japanese Rice

Makes 2–3 portions.
Fridge life: up to 4 days.

This is how I mostly cook rice, white with 'a handful' of other grains (and it's ok to add more than one handful, up to 2–3). Kombu and/or shiitake adds visual interest, extra nutients and little bites of flavour. Onigiri-friendly.

220g white Japanese rice
a handful of grains of your choice, like
   buckwheat, amaranth, oat groats,
   quinoa, millet, red rice or brown basmati
5cm piece of kombu seaweed and/or
   1 dried shiitake mushroom (stem
   broken off and discarded)
350ml water, to cook

Wash the combined grains with cold water directly in your cooking pot, trying to rub off as much of the cloudy starch as possible. Discard the water and repeat twice. Drain completely, push the kombu/shiitake into the rice and add the measured water for cooking.

→

Cover and bring to the boil, then simmer over a low heat for 15 minutes. Remove from the heat and leave to rest with the lid on for 5 minutes. Pick out the kombu and/or shiitake, cut into very thin strips then gently fold them back into the rice. Let it cool before packing in your bento and/or a storage container.

Black Gradient Rice

Makes 2–3 portions.
Fridge life: up to 4 days.

You often see a pinch of black rice added to white rice in Japanese home cooking, which gives it a soft lilac tint, with a slightly smoky flavour and chewy texture. The more black rice you add, the more dramatic the effect. Cooking 100% black is a little intense in flavour for everyday use I think (not to mention pricey), so I like to mix anything from a handful of black (= lilac rice) to half-half (= deep purple rice), getting a lot of colour out of one bag of black rice! Onigiri-friendly. →

Black gradient rice can be made with brown short-grain rice, too; just replace it for white in the measurements below, then proceed using the method for brown rice on page 30 (slow-cook or quick-cook both work well).

220g white Japanese rice
40g Venus black rice
400ml water, to cook

Wash the black and white rice combined with cold water directly in your cooking pot, trying to rub off as much of the cloudy starch as possible. Discard the water and repeat twice.

Drain completely and add the measured water for cooking. Cover and bring to the boil, then simmer over a low heat for 20 minutes.

Remove from the heat and leave to rest with the lid on for 5 minutes. Let it cool before packing in your bento and/or a storage container.

_____

Quinoa-sunflower Rice

Makes 2–3 portions.
Fridge life: up to 3 days.

Soft white rice is studded with specks of nutrient-rich quinoa and surprise sunflower seeds here. A light and soothing rice that goes with everything. Onigiri-friendly.

150g white Japanese rice
80g quinoa (black or red makes a nice
    visual contrast to the white rice)
2 tbsp sunflower seeds
350ml water, to cook

To add to the cooked grains:
½ tsp sea salt
1 tsp brown rice vinegar →

Wash the combined grains with cold water directly in your cooking pot, trying to rub off as much of the cloudy starch as possible. Discard the water and repeat once.

Drain completely and add the measured water for cooking. Cover and bring to the boil, then simmer over a low heat for 15 minutes.

Remove from heat and leave to rest with the lid on for 5 minutes. While still hot, fold in the salt and vinegar, taking care not to crush the grains too much. Let it cool before packing in your bento and/or a storage container.

_____

50/50 Rice

Makes 2–3 portions.
Fridge life: up to 3 days.

Best of both worlds! Brown rice's nutritional power with the fast cooking time of white rice. Balanced, calm and mineralizing. Onigiri-friendly.

110g white Japanese rice
110g brown short-grain rice
5cm piece of kombu seaweed
350ml water, to cook

Wash the combined white and brown rice with cold water directly in your cooking pot, trying to rub off as much of the cloudy starch as possible. Discard the water and repeat twice.

Drain, push the kombu into the rice and add the measured water. Cover and bring to the boil, then simmer over a low heat for 20 minutes.

Remove from the heat and leave to rest with the lid on for 5 minutes. Pick the kombu out and mince finely, then gently fold it back into the rice. Let it cool before packing in your bento and/or a storage container.

Multi-multi Rice

Makes 3–4 portions.
Fridge life: up to 3 days.

Hearty, earthy and filling, this rice has it all. Bright pomegranate sparks are optional but amazing. You can either slow-cook (the tastiest), or quick-cook (still very tasty!). The slow-cook version is onigiri-friendly.

200g brown short-grain rice
4 tbsp (40g) dried mung beans
4 tbsp (40g) dried aduki beans
4g dried hijiki or dried arame seaweed
450ml water, to cook

To add to the cooked rice:
1 tsp sea salt
2 tbsp brown rice or apple cider vinegar
seeds of ¼ pomegranate, optional

Slow-cook version:
Wash the combined rice, beans and seaweed with cold water directly in your cooking pot. Drain completely and add the measured water for cooking. Cover and leave to soak overnight, or for at least 6 hours.

The next day, without draining or removing the lid, bring to the boil, then simmer over a low heat for 20 minutes.

Quick-cook version:
No need to wash the rice. Soak the combined rice and beans in boiling water (any amount), directly in your cooking pot, for 30 minutes. Drain completely, and add seaweed and the measured water for cooking, but use boiling water. Cover and bring to the boil, then simmer over a low heat for 30 minutes.

For both versions:
Remove from the heat and leave to rest with the lid on for 10 minutes. While still hot, fold in the salt and vinegar, taking care not to crush the grains too much. Leave to cool, then gently mix in the pomegranate seeds, if using.

One-pot Rice – A Small Meal in Itself

I started putting veggies in with my rice to get 'two for the price of one' – the same principle as the mixed-grain rice. I throw a bunch of roughly chopped (hard) veggies and some nutrient-and-flavour-boosting ingredients in, and have half my bento covered once the rice is done! Just add some raw veggies, protein and/or sprinkles/boosts with your one-pot rice and you're set. Or, use it with any of the bento recipes in this book. For the one-pot rices, I like adding salt to bring the flavour of the veggies out (whilst for purer rice I don't, as per the Japanese way).

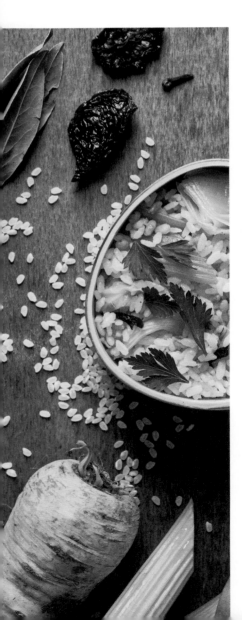

Farm Rice

Makes 2–4 portions.
Fridge life: up to 3 days.

This veggie selection is inspired by the clear, typically Swedish soups of my childhood and smells heavenly whilst cooking.

200g white Japanese rice
3 tbsp (30g) pearl barley or buckwheat
10cm piece of leek, 1 small carrot and
   1 stick celery, cleaned and cut into
   3cm pieces on the diagonal
3 sun-dried tomatoes, chopped
1 small bunch of flat-leaf parsley
1 dried bay leaf or 1 clove
½ tbsp extra virgin olive oil
1 tsp sea salt
350ml water, to cook

Wash the combined grains with cold water directly in your cooking pot, trying to rub off as much of the cloudy starch as possible. Discard the water and repeat twice.

   Drain completely, then pile the leek, carrot, celery, sun-dried tomatoes and the roughly chopped stalks of the parsley (save the leaves, chopped, to mix in with the cooked rice) on top of the rice – no need to mix them in. Push the bay leaf, or clove, into the rice and add the olive oil, salt and the measured water for cooking. Cover and bring to the boil, then simmer over a low heat for 15 minutes.

   Remove from the heat and leave to rest with the lid on for 5 minutes. Let it cool before packing in your bento and/or a storage container.

Happy Monk Rice

Makes 2–4 portions.
Fridge life: up to 3 days.

A sunshine-coloured rice with protein-boosting red lentils and mellow coconut. If you can, choose a squash with deep orange flesh, like kabocha or kuri (Hokkaido) squash. It is delicious eaten with colourful purple cabbage and broccoli quick-pickles (page 139) or with the Winter Jewel Salad Bento (page 122).

220g white Japanese rice
50g dried split red lentils
¼–½ small squash (200g prepped
   weight), peeled, deseeded and cut into
   bite-sized chunks
3 tbsp desiccated coconut
5cm piece of kombu seaweed
1 tsp sea salt
400ml water, to cook →

Wash the combined rice and lentils with cold water directly in your cooking pot, trying to rub off as much of the cloudy starch as possible. Discard the water and repeat twice.

Drain completely, stir in the squash and coconut, push the kombu into the rice and add the salt and the measured water for cooking. Cover and bring to the boil, then simmer over a low heat for 15 minutes.

Remove from the heat and leave to rest with the lid on for 5 minutes. Pick out the kombu and mince it finely, then gently fold it back into the rice. Let it cool before packing in your bento and/or a storage container.

Variation:
You can use carrot or sweet potato instead of squash. For a 'browner' version, use 170g white Japanese rice and 50g brown short-grain rice and proceed as above, but after removing from the heat, let it rest for 10 minutes.

Sister Power Rice

Makes 2–3 portions.
Fridge life: up to 3 days.

A real boost for our time of the month – all the ingredients are deeply mineralising (and pretty) and not just for women, of course, but for everyone! Try to use all the boosts if you can. To complete the cycle, try it with Lady Power Moon Bento on page 116. You can either slow-cook (the tastiest), or quick-cook (still very tasty!). The slow-cook version is onigiri-friendly. →

170g brown short-grain rice
50g dried aduki beans
1 small to medium beetroot, scrubbed and
    cut into bite-sized chunks
3 small dates (20g), roughly chopped
1 tsp sea salt
300ml water, to cook

Boosts for strength:

1 dried shiitake mushroom, stalk broken
    off and discarded, cap crumbled
3g dulse or ½ tsp instant dried wakame
1 tbsp raw cacao nibs
1 tbsp goji berries

Slow-cook version:

Wash the rice and beans with cold water directly in your cooking pot. Drain completely and add the beetroot, dates, salt and boosts, and measured water for cooking. Cover and leave to soak overnight or for at least 6 hours.

The next day, without draining or removing the lid, bring to the boil, then simmer over a low heat heat for 20 minutes.

Quick-cook version:

No need to wash the rice. Soak the rice and beans combined, in boiling water, directly in your cooking pot, for 30 minutes. Drain and add the beetroot, dates, salt and boosts, and measured water, but use boiling water. Cover and bring to the boil, then simmer over a low heat for 30 minutes.

For both versions:
Remove from the heat and leave to rest with the lid on for 10 minutes. Let it cool before packing in your bento and/or a storage container.

Sweet Gratitude Rice

Makes 2–3 portions.
Fridge life: up to 3 days.

This rice is a delight! Sweet, fragrant and soft and basmati makes a nice change to white Japanese rice. I'm even happy to eat it just as it is, with no extras!

150g white basmati rice
50g brown short-grain rice
3 dried figs, cut into bite-sized chunks
2 small firm apples, quartered and cored
    then halved
1 tbsp coconut oil (no need to melt it)
1 cardamom pod, broken
1 clove
½ tsp sea salt
350ml water, to cook

Wash both the basmati and brown rice combined with cold water directly in your cooking pot, trying to rub off as much of the cloudy starch as possible. Discard the water and repeat.

Drain completely, mix in the figs, apples, cardamom pod, clove, salt and measured water for cooking. Cover and bring to the boil, then simmer over a low heat for 15 minutes.

Remove from the heat and leave to rest with the lid on for 5 minutes. Let it cool before packing in your bento and/or a storage container.

Furikake – Seasoning / Nutrient Sprinkles

Furikake, seasoning sprinkles, is a favourite in Japanese households – an easy, instant way to perk up plain rice. Classic flavours are dry mixes of sesame seeds, seasoned seaweeds and dried fish, but there are also fresh kinds (kept in the fridge). Natural, additive-free furikake is difficult to find in the UK so I make my own! Sprinkle these over rice or noodles, or mix with warm rice to make onigiri. Delicious on toast too!

4–6 servings per nori sheet used.
Shelf life: up to 1 month.

Nori Confetti

A single-ingredient sprinkle with lots of flavour and mineral power! Nori is like paper, it can be cut into any shape, or folded and ripped into pieces.

To quickly make nori confetti for one bento, grab a nori sheet and fold it in half, then rip it, like paper. Use this half sheet (or halve again for less) per bento, and keep folding and ripping it apart over your bento – you can go down to quite small pieces like this.

To pre-prep confetti, fold one sheet in half, then carefully rip (or cut with scissors), fold again lenthways, and repeat until you have 8 long strips. Use sissors to cut the short end into the thinnest strips possible. Repeat with as many sheets as you like. Store in an airtight jar in your cupboard.

> *TIP:*
> To make an easy, classic furikake, mix nori confettis with gomashio, or with toasted sesame seeds and a little sea salt.

Makes 10–12 heaped tbsp servings.
Shelf life: up to 1 month.

Zen Pebble Furikake

A balanced all-rounder – neutral and crunchy, it goes with everything (even sprinkled over banana and honey toast!). Millet is a surprise ingredient here. Its flavour and yellow colour matches the freeze-dried egg yolk often found in ready-made (factory processed) furikake.

50g millet grain
50g black sesame seeds
½ tsp sea salt, dissolved in 1 tsp water (shake them together in a small container with a lid)
1 tbsp loose-leaf green sencha tea, optional

Toast the millet and sesame seeds in a dry frying pan over a medium heat, stirring occasionally to ensure the seeds don't burn. When they start to tan and release a slight smoke, 3–5 minutes, tip them to one side of the pan and quickly pour the salt water over, shaking the pan over the heat until the mix is completely dry.
Tip onto a plate and mix with the tea leaves, if using. Leave to cool completely, then pack in an airtight storage jar. Store in your cupboard.

Makes 10–12 ½ tbsp servings.
Fridge life: up to 1 week.

Wakame-san Fresh Furikake

Mixed with ginger, tamari and a little sweetness, mild-flavoured wakame seaweed is a classic flavour combo. Delicious mixed in with warm rice to make onigiri, as a topping on avocado or with quick-blanched/steamed greens.

1 tbsp dried instant wakame seaweed
3cm piece fresh ginger, washed but not peeled
½ tsp coconut palm sugar
1 tbsp tamari
1 tsp toasted white (hulled) sesame seeds

Place the seaweed in a bowl, cover with plenty of cold water and leave until soft and expanded (15 minutes). Drain, and squeeze in your hands to remove as much water as possible. Transfer to a chopping board and roughly chop. Finely grate the ginger.
Add the rehydrated wakame to a medium-hot pan and dry-fry, stirring more often as it gets drier and a little crunchy at the edges, 4–5 minutes. Then, push the wakame to one side of the pan, squeeze the grated ginger over it (discard the pulp), scatter the sugar over and finally add the tamari. Stir constantly until it looks drier but still a little moist, 1–2 minutes. Stir in the sesame seeds and tip onto a plate to cool completely, before storing in an airtight glass jar in the fridge.

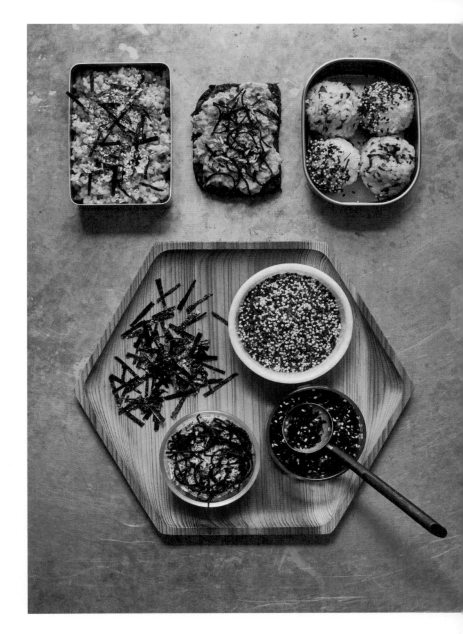

Makes 10–12 ½ tbsp servings.
Fridge life: up to 1 week.

Tao Beach Fresh Furikake

*Flavours from the sea with tangy
lime, coconut and a hot kick, with
all the nutritional goodness of hijiki.
This furikake instantly perks up plain
(white) rice, tofu and shredded chinese
cabbage. Yummy on avocado too!*

10g dried hijiki seaweed
30g desiccated coconut
1 tsp sea salt
1 tsp chilli flakes, or to taste
½ unwaxed lime

Place the seaweed in a bowl, cover
with plenty of cold water and leave
until soft and expanded, 15–20 minutes.
Drain. If the seaweed strands look like
they will be too long to eat comfortably,
chop them roughly.

Preheat a dry frying pan over a low
to medium heat and toast the coconut,
stirring until it has a slight tan, 1–2
minutes, then tip onto a plate.

Add the rehydrated hijiki and salt
to the hot pan and dry-fry, stirring
frequently over a medium heat until the
mixture is not soaking wet anymore,
4–5 minutes. Add the chilli flakes and
finely grate the lime peel and squeeze
the lime juice over the mixture. Continue
stirring until it's not soaking wet but still
a little moist. Stir in the toasted coconut,
tip back onto the plate and leave to
cool completely before storing in an
airtight glass jar in the fridge.

1. *Nori Confetti*
2. *Zen Pebble Furikake*
3. *Wakame-san Furikake*
4. *Tao Beach Furikake*

Gomashio – Sesame Salt

———

A little different from furikake, but sprinkled over noodles and rice in the same way, gomashio is toasted sesame seeds crushed with natural salt. I use it both as a 'flavour enhancer' (and not just for Asian foods, you could say it's a little like Parmesan) and as a way of boosting minerals and protein in my meals. Compared to typical recipes, my gomashio uses a lot less salt – simply so I can get more sesame in!

Use gomashio sprinkled over noodles and rice, just like furikake. Or, toss quick-blanched or shredded veggies in it for an instant side dish (or simply dump a spoonful on top of veggies directly in your bento). Use it as a kind of 'dry dressing' in salads, with avocado (adding fats, saltiness and flavour) or add a couple of spoonfuls to egg or seed omelettes. Best stored in the fridge as the oils in the crushed seeds are sensitive to heat.

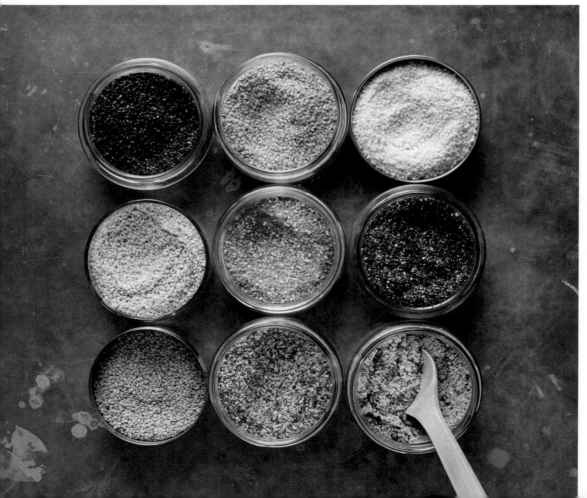

1. Black Toasted Sesame
2. Whole (unhulled) Gomashio
3. White (hulled) Gomashio
4. White (hulled) Toasted Sesame
5. Red Gomashio
6. Black Gomashio
7. Whole (unhulled) Toasted Sesame
8. Green Gomashio
9. Dulse Gomashio

Toasted Sesame Seeds

If I have just ONE sprinkle prepped and ready to go, this is the one. You'll notice it in many of my recipes and images and for a good reason: it couldn't be simpler to make or more versatile, adding flavour, slight crunch, nutritional value and good looks in a tiny sprinkle or a generous spoonful.

75g sesame seeds, any type: white (hulled), whole (unhulled) or black

Toast the sesame seeds in a dry frying pan over a low to medium heat, stirring occasionally to ensure they don't burn.
   When fragrant and starting to tan, 3–5 minutes, tip onto a plate and leave to cool completely before packing in an airtight storage jar. Store in your cupboard.

Each recipe makes
8–10 tbsp servings.
Fridge life: up to 1 month.

For all three gomashio options:

Toast the sesame seeds (plus pumpkin seeds for green gomashio) in a dry frying pan over low to medium heat, stirring occasionally to ensure the seeds don't burn. When fragrant, popping and starting to tan, 2–4 minutes, tip onto a plate and leave to cool completely.
   Add the seeds, seasonings and salt to a blender, and pulse, taking care not to over-blend. You should still be able to see a few whole sesame seeds in the mixture. Or, use a pestle and mortar to crush the seeds and salt, then mix the other ingredients in after (you will have to finely shred the nori sheet by hand if using this method). Store in an airtight glass jar in the fridge.

Black or White Gomashio

75g sesame seeds, white (hulled), whole (unhulled) or black
½ tsp rock or sea salt

Red Gomashio ('Chorizo')

Classic, super-savoury flavours in powder form! Perfect with Summer Fruits Bento (page 108) or on fresh tomatoes or peppers in your bento.

75g sesame seeds, white (hulled) or whole (unhulled)
1 tsp coconut palm sugar
2 tsp sweet smoked paprika
chilli flakes, to taste
½ tsp garlic granules, optional
1 tsp rock or sea salt

Green Gomashio ('Seafood')

The goodness of the sea along with some extra nutrients from pumpkin seed adds balance to eggs (sprinkle on sesame-fried egg whilst in the pan, or on halved overnight eggs), green peppers or green beans, and avocado.

50g sesame seeds, white (hulled) or whole (unhulled)
30g pumpkin seeds
2 tbsp aonori seaweed or 1½ sheets of nori, torn into stamp-sized pieces
½ tsp rock or sea salt

TIP:
I make my gomashio in the spice mill attachment on my Magimix blender. If you have a large blender, you may need to double these recipes for the seeds to crush properly.

Dulse Gomashio (Mineral and Umami Booster)

An all-round booster of both minerals and flavour for any food! I've soaked the sesame overnight here which brings a light, creamy flavour to the seeds (whole sesame can be a little bitter otherwise), as well as unlocking nutrients that are less available to us while the seeds are in 'hibernation'. You can make it with dried seeds too.

75g whole (unhulled) sesame seeds
10g dried dulse seaweed, roughly torn or cut with scissors into stamp-sized pieces
¼ tsp sea salt

If you have time, soak the sesame seeds in cold water overnight to then rinse and drain well in a strainer.
   Preheat a dry frying pan over a low to medium heat, then add the dulse and toast until completely brittle, about 5 minutes. Move the dulse around occasionally to prevent burning. Tip onto a plate.
   Add the drained, wet sesame seeds to the hot pan and toast, stirring more frequently as they become drier to ensure they don't burn. When they are very fragrant, look completely dry and a little puffed up, 10–15 minutes if done from wet, 3–5 minutes from dry, tip onto a plate and leave to cool.
   Add to a (small) blender, pulse the cool sesame seeds, dulse and salt, just until the mixture starts looking a little moist. Store in an airtight glass jar in the fridge.

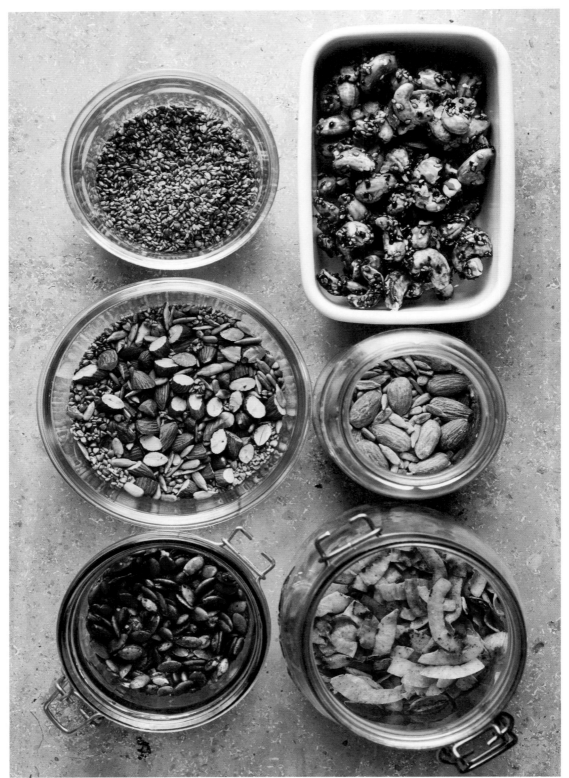

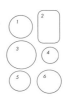

1. Tamari Seeds
2. Cashew Nut
   Clusters
3. Savoury Granol[e]
4. Saltwater-toaste[d]
   Nuts and Seeds
5. Chilli-toasted
   Pumpkin Seeds
6. Coconut 'Fakeo[n]

Seasoned Nuts and Seeds

Seasoned nuts and seeds make quick, savoury boosts of proteins and whole fats to a bento and they are low-maintenace – just prep a batch and enjoy for weeks (I usually double or even triple these recipes). Either add directly to your bento or pack in a small separate container (to keep them crunchy). Don't be shy to use these nuts and seeds by the handful – they bring filling power and essential nutrients to your bento (and your day)!

Makes 10–15 heaped tbsp servings.
Shelf life: 1 month or more.

1. Savoury Granola

If you manage not to eat all of this right after making it, it is delicious on everything from leafy greens to filling onigiri with (page 114). Sprinkle generously!

75g whole almonds, roughly chopped
25g buckwheat and/or sunflower seeds
25g sesame seeds (any type)
1 tbsp coconut palm sugar
½ tsp flaky sea salt
a pinch of chilli flakes

Variations:
In addition to the ingredients above, add either one, or both, of the following: pinch of dried rosemary, a few fine grates of organic lemon zest

Toast the nuts, grains and seeds in a dry frying pan over a low to medium heat, stirring occasionally to ensure they don't burn. When very fragrant and starting to tan, 4–6 minutes, tip the mixture to one side of the pan and scatter over the sugar, salt and other flavourings, if using. Stir briefly until the sugar has melted.

  Tip onto a plate, then leave to cool completely before storing in an airtight jar in your cupboard.

Makes 10–15 heaped tbsp servings.
Shelf life: up to 2 weeks.

2. Cashew Nut Clusters

A few of these salty-sweet hunks are gold to any bento. You can use any other nuts mixed with, or in place of, the cashews.

1 tbsp maple syrup or 1½ tbsp coconut palm sugar dissolved in 1 tbsp hot water
½ tbsp tamari
½ tbsp fresh lemon juice
100g cashews
1 tbsp each of white (hulled) and black sesame seeds
¼ tsp flaky sea salt, smoked if possible

Mix the syrup, tamari and lemon juice in a small glass. Toast the nuts in a dry frying pan over a low to medium heat, stirring occasionally to ensure they don't burn. When the nuts start looking a little tanned, 2–3 minutes, add the sesame seeds and toast for a few more moments, stirring frequently until the seeds pop a lot and have a litle colour. Tip the mixture to one side of the pan and quickly drizzle the syrup mix over, stirring with a wooden spoon over the heat until the moisture has evaporated. Sprinkle the salt over and stir in. Tip onto a sheet of baking paper, then leave to cool completely before breaking in chunks and storing in an airtight jar in your cupboard.

Makes 10–15 heaped tbsp servings.
Shelf life: up to 2 weeks.

3. Coconut 'Fakeon'

Crispy, smoky, oily, and irresistible – top anything with these, or mix with sultanas, dried bilberries or dates for a sweet-savoury snack to take away. Makes a great drinks snack too. Just saying!

60g dried coconut flakes (chips)
1 tsp coconut palm sugar
½ tsp smoked paprika
½ tsp sea salt
a pinch each of garlic granules and chilli flakes, optional

Gently toast the coconut flakes in a dry frying pan over a low to medium heat, stirring all the time with a wooden spoon to ensure they don't burn. When they start browning, scatter all the seasonings over, stir to mix thoroughly, and toast for a few more moments to allow the sugar to melt.

  Tip onto a plate, then leave to cool completely before storing in an airtight jar in your cupboard.

Savoury Toasted Nuts and Seeds

If you ever wondered how to get seasoning to stick to toasted nuts like the ones you buy in shops, this is how! Simply douse your hot, toasted nuts in a salty seasoning liquid and let it evaporate away for a few moments over the heat in your pan – the seasoning will stick to the nuts. The liquid can be varied endlessly; I've included a few variations here to get you going.

Saltwater-toasted Nuts and Seeds

These are my staple 'cupboard proteins' for bento: you only need nuts, salt, water and a frying pan to have them ready in minutes. Liquid smoke, a natural seasoning which adds a smokey flavour really takes them next level ('nut bacon', anyone?) or experiment with dried herbs or ground spices added to your saltwater mix. Great mixed with sultanas as a snack on the side.

a little under ½ tsp sea salt
1 tbsp water
¼ tsp liquid smoke seasoning, optional
125g mixed whole almonds and
 sunflower seeds

All recipes make 10–15
heaped tbsp servings.
Shelf life: 1 month or more.

Tamari Seeds

Flavourful sesame and linseeds combined with crunchy buckwheat here, making a delicious pretty finishing sprinkle in your bento, especially good on sweet ingredients.

1 tsp tamari
1 tsp water
50g sesame seeds (any type)
25g linseeds
25g buckwheat

Chilli-toasted Pumpkin Seeds

Adjust the heat to your own liking for nuggets of fire to sprinkle over anything and everything!

a little under ½ tsp sea salt
1 tsp chilli powder, or to taste
 (I like chipotle)
pinch of garlic granules, optional
1 tbsp water
125g pumpkin seeds

For all three options:

Make the salty seasoning liquid: Shake the salt and water, or tamari and water, plus any flavourings, together in a small jar with a lid.

Toast the nuts/seeds/grains in a dry frying pan over a low to medium heat, stirring occasionally to ensure they don't burn.

When the nuts/seeds/grains are very fragrant and starting to tan, 2–4 minutes, tip them to one side of the pan and quickly drizzle the seasoning liquid over, stirring with a wooden spoon until they look completely dry, about 1 minute. (Tipping them over to one side like this – piling them into a thick layer – ensures more of the nuts/seeds/grains catch the liquid before it gets lost to the base of the pan.)

Tip onto a plate and leave to cool completely before storing in an airtight jar in your cupboard.

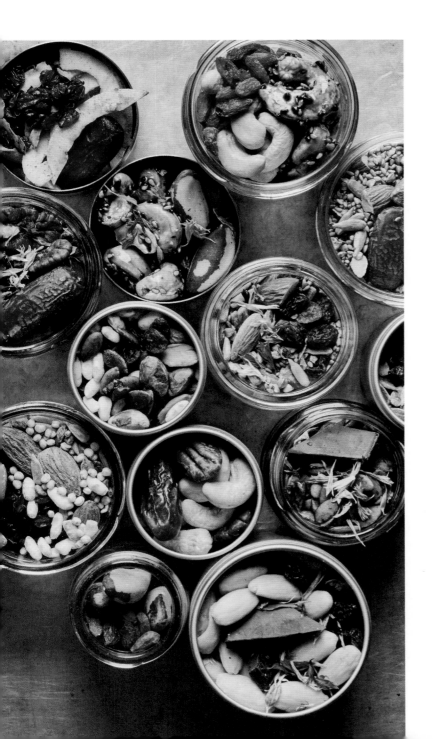

Little Pots of Tricks

However convenient it is to grab a bag of nuts while on the go, it adds to that personal mountain of trash (built over a lifetime) and you pay a premium for someone else packing your nuts! So, I try to play snack-factory as often as I can – I open up all the small (repurposed) containers my kitchen overflows with and fill them with whatever I have at hand. Seasoned nuts and seeds are star fillers! Either make a big mix and fill your pots or make each pot a little different for a surprise. Those ready-packed, overpriced snacks can go and sulk in the corner.

Inside the pots:
Cashews, pecans, brazils, blanched
　　almonds
Dates, sultanas, barberries (sour and
　　amazing), goji berries
Raw cacao nibs
Dark chocolate
Savoury granola
Cashew nut clusters
Coconut 'Fakeon'
Saltwater-toasted nuts and seeds
Chilli-toasted pumpkin seeds
Gluten-free Mighty Muesli (page 57)
Dried cornflower petals just for fun!

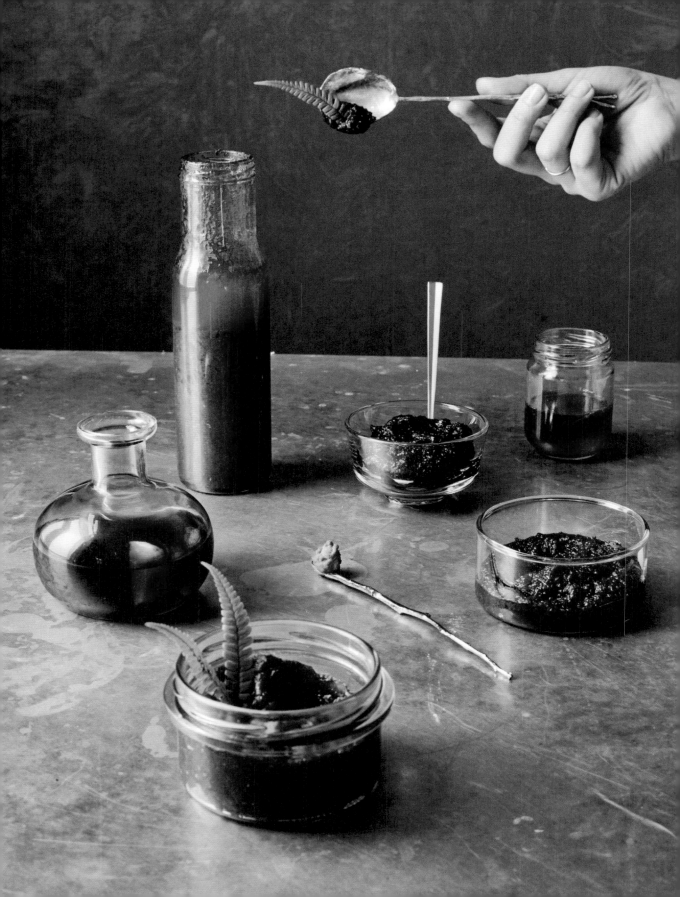

Liquid Seasoning Potions

All these potions are easy to put together, last for ages and transform a simple bento (or any meal) into something special with just one or two spoonfuls. In my kitchen, nothing is 'just' seasonings alone, so all these (apart from the wasabi) double up as 'nutrient potions' too!

Makes 50ml.
Fridge life: several months.

Garlic-infused Soy Sauce

This super-simple seasoning adds instant oomph and can be used in place of tamari in any of the recipes in this book. There's a lot of power in one garlic clove, so I usually keep mine a few months and just top up with fresh tamari as my bottle runs low.

50ml tamari
1 garlic clove, peeled and halved lengthways

Add the tamari and garlic to a small, repurposed bottle (ideally one with a pouring cap/top), close and refrigerate. It's ready to use after a day or so. The flavour deepens over time.

Makes about 6 tbsp servings (although you may want to use more than 1 tbsp per serving). Fridge life: up to 2 weeks.

Korean-style Dressing

I often make this dressing in my bento workshops and the moment people try it, they get hooked on gochugaru – Korean red pepper (and on the dressing too, I think!). Mixed with rice vermicelli or plain rice it makes it deliciously orangey-red. If you can't source gochugaru, the substitute mix is very tasty too!

1 tbsp gochugaru (Korean red pepper) (see Substitute mix)
1 tbsp coconut palm sugar
1½ tbsps brown rice vinegar
½ tbsp tamari
3 tbsps toasted sesame oil (see Tip)
1 tsp fine sea salt
½ tsp garlic granules, optional

Pour all the ingredients into a small glass jar with a lid and give it a really good shake. Store in the fridge, and shake well before using.

Substitute mix
Sub the gochugaru with 1 tsp chilli flakes, 1 tsp paprika and 1 tsp sweet smoked paprika, combined.

TIP:
Double, triple, quadruple these recipes – it will take the same amount of time to prepare, is really handy to have on hand and keeps well (apart from the wasabi).

TIP:
Korean style dressing: If you like to save on your toasted sesame oil, replace up to half of its volume with a light oil like grapeseed oil or cold-pressed sesame oil.

Makes 6 tbsp servings.
Fridge life: up to 1 month.

Cheatin' Gochujang Sauce

Gochujang is a seasoning paste essential in many Korean dishes – it goes with everything and is simply addictive! You may know it as the spicy, sweet sauce served with Bibimbap. I spent years looking for one that wasn't full of flavour enhancers or corn syrup – in the end I made my own.

Original gochujang needs fermenting for months, but I don't have the patience (or skill). To create mine, I used something that's already fermented – miso paste – then added the signature gochujang flavours. I've excluded garlic in my version to keep it meeting-friendly but you can add grated fresh garlic or garlic granules to taste, if you like.

I use gochujang as a quick enhancer for any rice- or noodle-based bento (just add a dollop and let each person mix it into their food), or 1–2 spoonfuls as a quick marinade/dressing for veggies (try it with cucumber and cauliflower). It's also amazing spread on toast with almond butter, smoked tofu or avocado!

2 tbsp gochugaru (Korean red pepper) or
   1 tsp each of chilli flakes, paprika and
   sweet smoked paprika
2 tbsp brown rice miso paste
2 tbsp brown rice syrup or
   1 tbsp agave syrup
1 tbsp tamari
1 tbsp toasted sesame oil, optional

In a small storage jar with a lid, mix all the ingredients to a very smooth paste. Store in the fridge.

Variation: Different types of miso give different results. I love the darker misos for this recipe.

Makes 10 tsp servings.
Fridge life: 2 months or more.

Lazy Ra-yu Chilli Oil

Ra-yu is a spicy sesame oil typically used to spice up Chinese-origin dishes like ramen or dumplings. Here is a lazy version, skipping on the steps but hopefully not on flavour. Use as a quick boost to overnight boiled eggs (which can be a little hard and dry), drizzled over rice or noodles, onigiri or quick-blanched greens.

50ml toasted sesame oil
5cm piece of leek, cleaned and very
   thinly sliced
2cm piece fresh ginger, washed but not
   peeled, finely grated
2 tbsp gochugaru (Korean red pepper) or
   2 tsp each of chilli flakes, paprika and
   sweet smoked paprika
grated zest of ¼ unwaxed lemon
1 small dried chilli pepper, to soak in the
   bottle, optional

Gently heat the oil in a small pan. When it starts looking hot, drop the leek and ginger into it – it will bubble and fizz. Once that has calmed down, remove it from the heat and stir in the rest of the ingredients.

Leave to cool, then strain through a fine sieve (I use a metal tea strainer) into a small, repurposed glass jar or bottle, ideally one with a pouring cap. Add the dried chilli, if using, and seal and store in the fridge.

Makes about 7 tbsp servings.
Fridge life: up to 1 month.

Miso Almond Seasoning Paste

A very moreish combination of flavours. Great as an onigiri filler, or add a blob into your bento and eat with plain rice or veggies. Dilute a couple of tablespoons with a little water to make a delicious noodle dressing. You can use tahini or peanut butter instead of almond.

3 tbsp almond butter
3 tbsp brown rice miso paste
½ tbsp maple syrup

Flavour options (add one of these to the mixture above):
a little finely grated unwaxed lemon zest
   and 2 tbsp lemon juice
1 tsp gochugaru (Korean red pepper) or
   chilli flakes, to taste
5cm piece fresh ginger, grated and juice
   hand-squeezed out (pulp discarded)

Mix all the ingredients to a very smooth paste directly in a small storage jar with a lid. Store in the fridge.

Makes 1–2 servings.
Use the same day.

Wasabi from Powder

I was taught the very simple art of making wasabi from powder working in a Stockholm sushi restaurant as a student. Wasabi's pungency is volatile, so you want to stop it from disappearing into the air. Solution: trap it in an upside-down glass.

1 tsp wasabi powder
½ tsp water
pinch of sea salt

Stir the wasabi powder and water together in a small glass to a paste. Leave the glass upside-down (the paste should be sticking to the 'roof' of the glass) to allow the pungency to develop for at least 5 minutes.

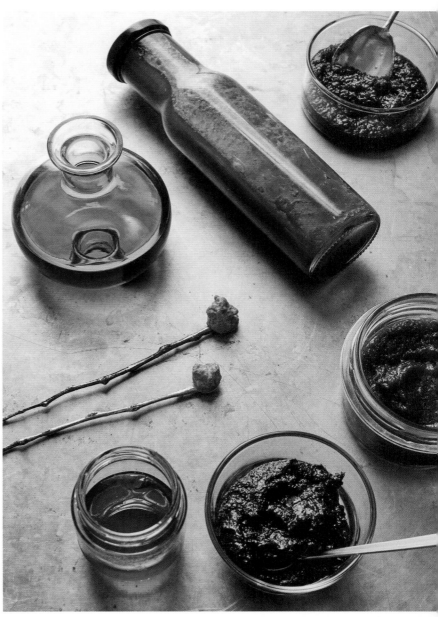

1. Garlic-infused Soy Sauce
2. Korean-style Dressing
3a. Gochujang (made with brown rice miso)
3b. Gochujang (made with hatcho miso)
4. Lazy Ra-yu Chilli Oil
5. Miso Almond Seasoning Paste
6. Wasabi from Powder

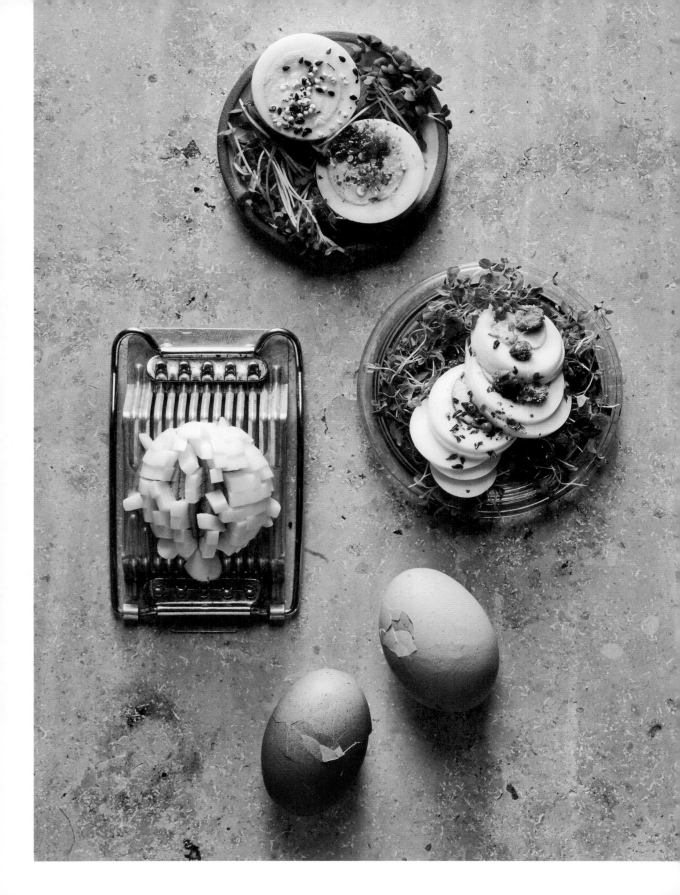

Overnight Eggs

Overnight eggs are all about getting fast, tasty proteins into your bento, with as little preparation as possible. Even when I'm absolutely knackered and ready for bed, I can still fill up a pot of eggs for tomorrow's bento and let them get ready overnight. The technique is (very) loosely based on the Japanese tradition of cooking eggs in natural hot springs for several hours over a low heat. The only tiny drawback is that these become very well done (= dry), but that's easy to remedy with seasonings; my tried-and-tested favourites are here.

Makes as many as you like.
Fridge life: up 5 days (unpeeled).

For the overnight eggs:
As many organic eggs as you like, medium or large

Before going to bed, place the eggs in the smallest cooking pan they will fit into and *just* cover them with water. Cover with a lid and bring to the boil, then immediately turn the heat off. Without removing the lid, leave until the morning when they're ready to drain (see Tip), peel and pack, or store (unpeeled) in the fridge for later use.

Easy peel hack: In the morning, change the water in the pan (just to be on the safe side), then drop the eggs into the pan so they crack against its base. Leave in the water for a minute or so, then it's easy to lift rather than 'scratch' the peel off (don't do this if you plan to store the eggs though).

> TIP:
> Houseplants LOVE egg cooking water! Rather than draining into the sink, give it straight to your plants (never water plants with hot or warm water).

Egg Cuts

Halved:

Simplest possible! Cut in half widthways so you get 2 round rather than oval shapes (for visual effect, and compactness), and place both halves, yolk-up, in your bento. Top with any of the seasonings.

Sliced:

If you plan on getting serious about hard-boiled eggs in bento, get an egg slicer (I grew up with the kind in the image). It will quickly get your egg into easy-to-eat slices, to spread over rice or in a salad.

Pixelated:

A level up from sliced! Slice the egg once (in your egg slicer), then turn it 90 degrees and gently slice again and you have pixels. Not just cute, but this is the optimal way to get your egg to absorb as much of the liquid seasoning as possible.

Pixelated and mixed in with rice:

For a satisfying egg-not-fried-rice, pixelate (or mash with a fork) your egg straight into your empty box, mix with your rice and optional seasonings, then push the rice to one side and fill up the rest with your veggies and sides.

Egg Seasonings

By lunchtime the egg should be slightly 'marinated' in the seasonings you have topped them with and any excess will have seeped into the rice, flavouring it further.

Try one of these seasonings:
a little toasted sesame oil + a sprinkle of sea salt or tamari
a little Lazy Ra-yu chilli oil (page 48) + a sprinkle of sea salt
a little of your favourite hot chilli sauce + sprinkle of sea salt
a little garlic infused-soy sauce (page 47)
a little tamari + furikake or chilli flakes
a little flaxseed oil + a sprinkle of sea salt + celery or cumin seed
Salted capers + a little extra virgin olive oil
a little tamari + aonori seaweed

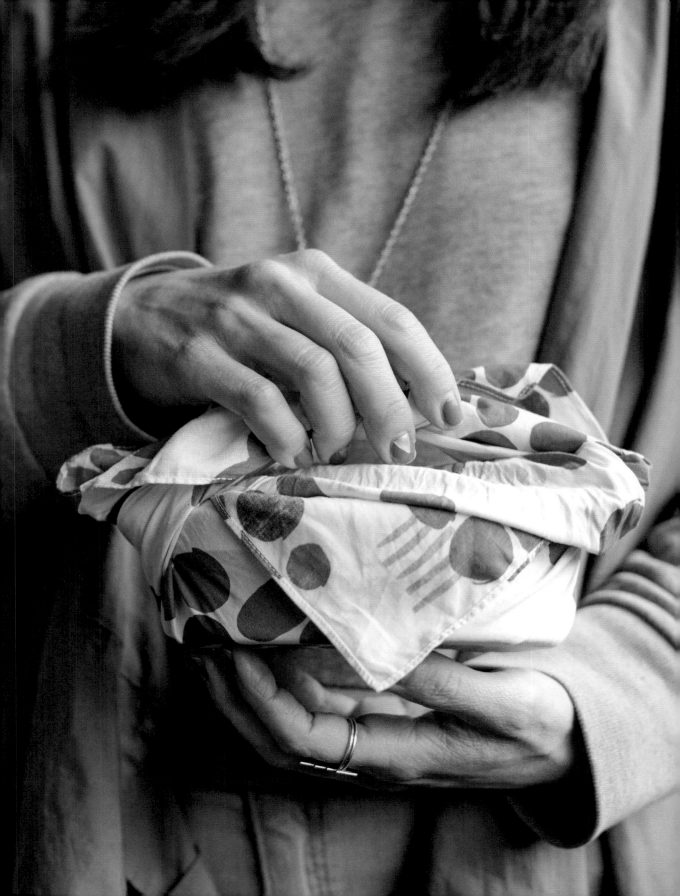

BREAKFAST and SWEET BENTO

Charge the start of your day and your break time with some of my most loved breakfast and snack recipes, just as good eaten at home as taken away. The roots of these recipes are from my Scandinavian background, powered-up with ingredients, flavours and ideas I've fallen in love with along the way.

Breakfast Bulk-blends

I love making breakfast blends in bulk. Just one burst of prep and then you can enjoy days, weeks even, without any decisions or hassle in the mornings (I'm not a morning person). I grew up with muesli or oats in the morning – my doctor parents' idea of a healthy breakfast. When I first met Andy, I was amazed at the amount of (overpriced and over-packed) muesli he went through every week, so I started getting ingredients in bulk to make our own. Here are our favourites! The recipes roughly amount to a packet of supermarket cereal; personally, I'd at least double or even quadruple the amounts (which means more decision-free mornings!).

Sesame Snap Granola

This granola happened while on a family holiday on a small island where the only tiny supermarket stocked basics including sesame seeds and olive oil. Luckily, I'd brought rice syrup (some type of syrup is essential for the granola to lump together, and yes I always travel with ingredients!) and Sesame Snap Granola was born. After my random discovery, this recipe has been on repeat in our house. To make it go further, I like mixing 2 parts ready granola with 1 part rolled jumbo oats and 1 part dried fruit (sultanas).

Makes about 450g
(8–10 servings).
Shelf life: up to 1 month.
Freezer life: up to 2 months.

150g rolled oats
100g sesame seeds (any type)
40g desiccated coconut
75g almonds and/or brazil nuts or
  pecans, whole or roughly chopped
3 tbsp (35g) flaxseeds
2 tbsp (20g) extra virgin olive oil
4 tbsp (50g) brown rice syrup

Preheat the oven to 150°C/300°F/ gas mark 2 and line a large baking tray with baking paper. Add all the ingredients to a large mixing bowl (see Tip) and thoroughly mix them together. Spread the mixture evenly over the tray and bake for 30 minutes, until tanned but not dark. Stir every 10 minutes to ensure the mixture doesn't burn. If you've doubled the recipe, bake for another 10–15 minutes. To get bigger clusters, gather the hot granola together in a pile (once it's out of the oven) before letting it cool completely on the baking paper. Transfer the mix to an airtight storage jar.

TIP:
If you have digital kitchen scales, there's a hack to zoom through the ingredients list in no time: place the empty bowl on to the scales and set to zero. Add one ingredient at a time, and reset the scales to zero between each addition.

TIP:
My friend Heike of Tasty as Heck taught me to keep granola in the freezer – not only to make it last longer, but to make it incredibly crunchy if eaten right away from frozen!

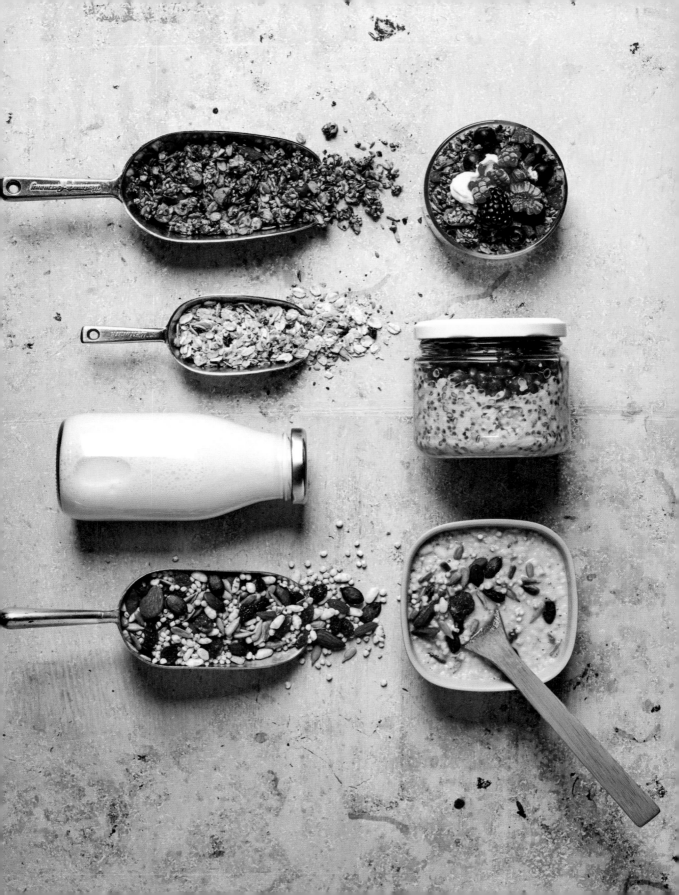

Scoop-and-go Overnight Mix

Overnight oats are one of our favourite breakfasts! I like making a big batch of ready-to-scoop mix packed full of nutritious, filling seeds and ground almonds that act as a sort of instant nut milk. Activate with water or plant-based milk overnight (try the Happy-powered Hemp Milk on page 60). I like adding a spoonful of honey (small-scale produced) to the mix when I soak it overnight and sometimes a drizzle of flaxseed oil too, for extra power. Keep the dry mix in the fridge to protect the ingredients' delicate oils.

600g rolled jumbo oats
75g sunflower or pumpkin seeds
50g chia seeds
50g linseeds
50g almond flour (aka ground almonds
  – see Tip)
75g hulled hemp seeds (if your diet is
  plant-based, use 150g for extra protein)
2 tbsp raw cacao nibs or raw
  cacao powder

Makes 900g (10–15 servings).
Fridge life: up to 1 month.

Combine all the ingredients in a large mixing bowl or directly in a big storage container with a lid and mix well. Transfer to storage (if it's not already in one) and store in the fridge.

To activate:
If I'm taking my oats with me, I like using a re-purposed glass jar with screw on lid, like in the image. In the evening before you want to serve the oats (or, in the morning before taking it as a snack to work), add cold water or plant-based milk (the mixture will expand about 1.5 times in volume, so be generous with the liquid) and any extras like honey or fruit. Stir to release the milkiness, cover and leave overnight. I prefer to eat the oats at room temperature, so I leave them out overnight (unless the weather is very hot), but you can leave them in the fridge if you prefer.

TIP:
If you can't find almond flour (aka ground almonds), blitz blanched almonds or cashews in your blender to make flour.

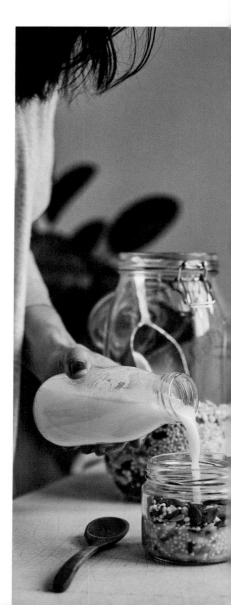

Gluten-free Mighty Muesli

Here's a gluten (and oat) free muesli, based on affordable sunflower seeds and sultanas, made extraordinary by adding lemon zest, puffed grains and a handful of unusual dried fruit. Eaten with hemp milk (see page 60) this muesli is both light and filling and became an obsession for a while when writing this book. This muesli adds filling power as a topping for smoothies too – and is great eaten by the handful as a pick-me-up!

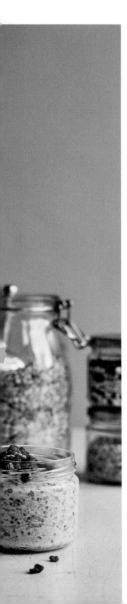

Makes 550g (8–10 portions).
Shelf life: up to 2 months.

150g sunflower seeds
50g pumpkin seeds
50g whole almonds
200g sultanas
zest of ½ unwaxed lemon, finely grated
50g puffed quinoa (see Tip)
25g puffed brown rice
25g interesting dried fruit (like goji berries, inca berries, mulberries)

Start by toasting the seeds and almonds, either in a frying pan or the oven (see Tip). To pan-toast, add the seeds and almonds to a dry frying pan over a low to medium heat and stir occasionally until they're fragrant and a little tanned, about 5 minutes. To oven-toast, preheat the grill to medium-high and spread the seeds and almonds evenly over a large baking tray, then toast them high up in the oven, stirring a few times until fragrant and a little tanned, about 10 minutes. Watch them closely to ensure they don't burn.

While the seeds and almonds toast, place the sultanas in a big mixing bowl, or directly in a big storage container, and finely grate the lemon zest over.

As soon as the seeds and almonds are toasted, add them *hot* to the sultanas and zest and combine. Their heat releases the aromatic oils from the zest, which infuses with the rest of the ingredients. The heat also livens up the dried fruit and dehydrates the zest (so there's no risk it will spoil). Leave the mixture to cool before adding the rest of the ingredients and combine. Transfer to storage if it's not already in one, ensuring it is fully cool before closing as condensation will spoil the muesli.

TIPS:
Puffed quinoa is worth tracking down for its interesting looks alone (not to mention texture and nutritional value). It's more than double the price at a regular supermarket compared to online, so get bulk-shopping!

Oven-toasting is more practical if you are doubling or quadrupling the recipe (which I tend to do).

Savoury Banana Bread

———

I'm always on the look-out for snacks that are not too sweet, but still have that instant pick-me-up effect in the afternoon (or late morning, or late at night!) and this unique banana bread ticks all of those boxes. It's flour-free, only sweetened with bananas and sultanas and full of the power of nuts, seeds – and seaweed! I've used miso paste and ginger for a rounded, satisfying flavour. It's seriously good spread with avocado or nut butter and toasted it's next level!

Makes 1 loaf (5–8 portions).
Fridge life: up to 5 days.
Freezer life: up to 1 month.

Dry ingredients

50g rolled jumbo oats
50g almonds (blanched or whole)
50g sunflower seeds
1 ½ tsp baking powder
60g raisins
10g hijiki seaweed

Wet ingredients

3 ripe bananas (300g peeled weight) +
    1 to decorate, cut lengthways
100ml water
1 tbsp brown rice miso
4cm piece fresh ginger, finely grated,
    juice hand-squeezed straight into the
    mix (pulp discarded)

Preheat the oven to 180°C/350°F/gas mark 4. Line a 20 x 10 cm loaf tin with baking paper.

Put the dry ingredients, apart from the raisins and seaweed into a blender (or a food processor) and blend to make a coarse flour. Transfer to a bowl and mix in the raisins and seaweed. Without washing your blender out (or food processor), blend all the wet ingredients together until smooth. Gently fold the wet mixture into the dry mix, to a loose porridge consistency. Take care not to mix it too much, so leave some lumps of flour in.

Pour into the loaf tin and carefully lay the banana halves on top. Bake for 30–35 minutes until the bread doesn't wobble when prodding the tin – it's better slightly under-baked than over-baked.

Remove from the oven and cover with a clean tea towel, then turn the loaf upside down in the tin to keep the moisture in and leave it to cool completely on a board. Once cool, cut into slices or bite-sized squares to serve. Store wrapped airtight in the fridge.

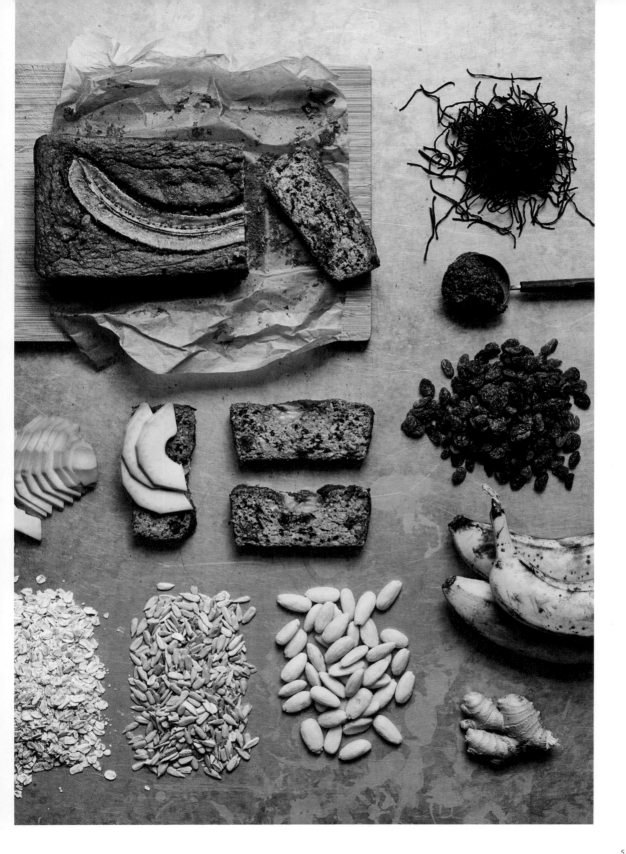

Happy-powered Hemp Milk

There's no going back now that I've discovered just how good home-made hemp milk is. It ticks all my boxes for a star everyday food: delicious (although some may find hemp tastes unusual to begin with), really easy to make (just blend with water, no soaking, no straining, no waste!), nutritious, rich in protein (about a third of total weight) and essential fatty acids (also about a third), affordable and hemp is a crop that grows in Europe. Pure, happy plant power! I use it with Gluten-free Mighty Muesli (page 57), to soak the Scoop-and-go overnight mix in (page 56) or to make a matcha or black tea latte.

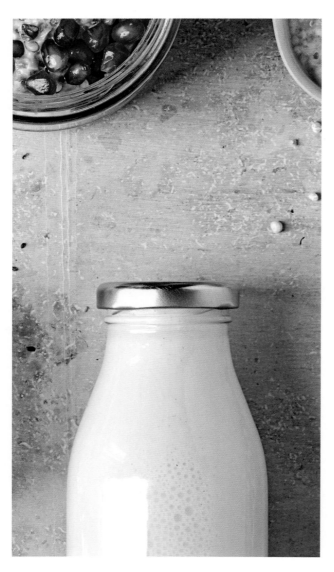

Makes about 500ml milk.
Fridge life: Up to 3 days.

500ml water
2 tbsp (20g) shelled hemp seeds
a pinch of sea salt
½ tbsp clear honey or maple syrup, or
   2 soft, small dates (20g), optional
a pinch of vanilla powder (Ndali whole
   ground vanilla pod is ideal) or a drop of
   natural vanilla extract, optional

In a blender, blend all the ingredients on the highest speed for at least 1 minute until completely smooth. Pour into a clean, repurposed glass bottle or jar with a lid and store in the fridge. Shake the milk before using as the seed sediments will settle.

Mood-boosting Cacao Balls

Only dates are used to sweeten these little feel-good balls and the speed of throwing them together is just as mood-boosting as their ingredients! The vitamin C in the optional pomegranate seeds helps your body to absorb iron, of which there's a lot of in raw cacao. You can also choose to finish by rolling them in desiccated coconut. I like raw coconut oil, but I don't always want my food to taste of it, so whenever I can I use odourless coconut oil instead (always organic).

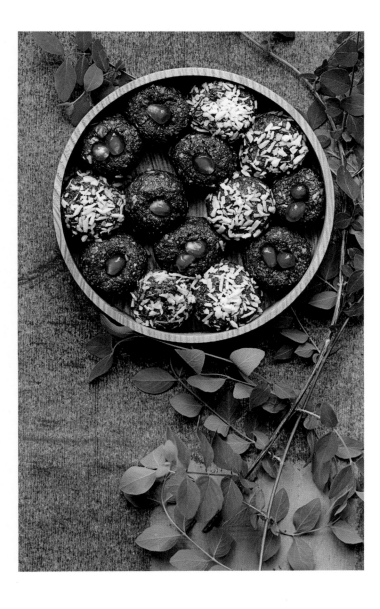

Makes about 12 x 3cm balls.
Fridge life: up to 2 weeks (excluding pomegranate seeds).

50g rolled jumbo oats
50g cashews
80g pitted soft dates (I use deglet nour)
3 tbsp raw cacao powder (or use regular unsweetened cocoa powder)
2 tbsp coconut oil, raw or organic odourless (no need to melt)
¼ tsp natural vanilla powder or extract (Ndali whole ground vanilla pod is ideal)
a good pinch of sea salt
pomegranate seeds, to garnish, optional

Put the oats and cashews in a blender and blend to a coarse flour. Tear or snip the dates in half using scissors, straight into the blender, and blend again to a coarse flour. Add the rest of the ingredients, apart from the pomegranate seeds, and pulse for a few moments until you have a sticky, handle-able dough. Roll into balls straight away and, if you like, press a few pomegranate seeds into each ball. Store in an airtight container in the fridge.

Fluffy Grain-free Pancakes with Overnight Chia Jam

At the start of my Instagram journey, I was amazed by the amount of pancakes people posted. Most were the small fluffy kind in a pretty stack with chocolate dribbling down its sides. I wanted some too! Somewhere I read you could make pancakes out of nuts and eggs and so I did. These little flourless wonders are packed with protein and good fats and are equally good with sweet or savoury toppings. Overnight chia jam is my little hack to have jam ready for breakfast with minimal effort. What is chia jam? I'd prefer to call it 'instant jam' with the benefits of gelatinous chia seed (hydrating, fibre, omegas) and being able to use any natural sugar I like.

Makes 12–16 tiny pancakes
(6cm diameter), 1–3 portions.
Fridge life pancakes and chia jam:
up to 3 days.
Freezer life (pancakes only):
up to 1 month.

Overnight Chia Jam

200g frozen raspberries
1 tbsp chia seeds
2 tbsp coconut palm sugar or
   1 tbsp clear honey, or to taste
4 tbsp water

The jam is best made the evening before you want to serve it, or at least 4 hours before, but you can do a speedy version too. Place all the ingredients in a glass jar with a lid, close and give it a good shake. As soon as the water touches the chia seeds they start swelling and sticking together, so if you can, shake the jar a couple of times during the first 30 minutes or so.

If you're making a speedy version, place your jar in a pan of hot water (to melt the berries) and it's ready to use after about an hour. For the overnight version, the berries will slowly melt and plump up the seeds with their juice. Give it another shake and taste to see if it's sweet enough; if not, add a little extra sugar or honey.

Cashew Pancakes

100g cashews
2 organic medium eggs
¼ tsp baking powder
pinch of sea salt
100ml water
a little oil, to fry

Place the cashews in a blender and blend to make a coarse flour, then add the rest of the ingredients (except the oil for frying) and blend on the highest setting until very thick and fluffy, like whipped custard – this will take a couple of minutes in a standard blender. Add a little more water if the mixture seems too thick to blend or pour.

Preheat a frying pan over a medium heat and rub with a little oil. Pour the batter straight out of the blender (or use a spoon) to form small pancakes in the pan (see Tip) and then lower the heat. (You'll need to cook the pancakes in batches.) When you start seeing small bubbles at the top of the pancakes, after about 1 minute, gently flip them over and cook for a further minute or so. Remove to a plate and cover with a piece of baking paper, then leave to cool before packing in your bento. Repeat to make the rest of the pancakes, until all the batter has been used up.

TIP:
To make the bear pancakes, once you've poured a dollop of batter in your pan for a pancake, use a small spoon and carefully drop a little batter at the edges of each pancake. Flip gently. For the eyes, melt a little dark chocolate either in a heat-proof bowl over a pan of simmering water, or in a microwave oven. Once the pancake is fully cool, draw the face on with a cocktail stick or very thin chopsticks.

   To freeze, ensure the pancakes are fully cool, then lay in one layer in a large ziplock bag – you can then take them out one at a time and heat in your toaster, or simply pack in your bento to defrost by lunchtime.

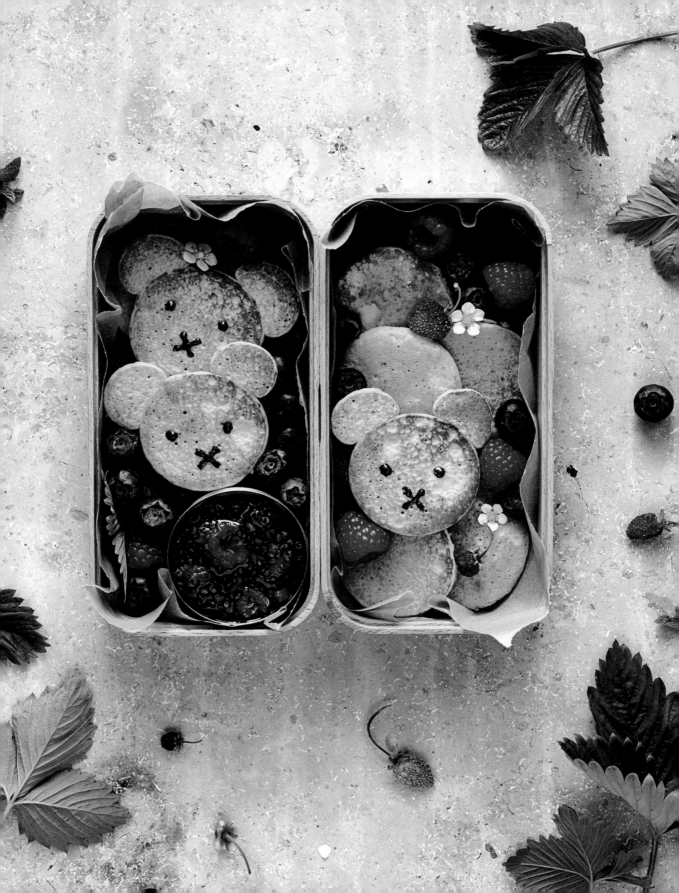

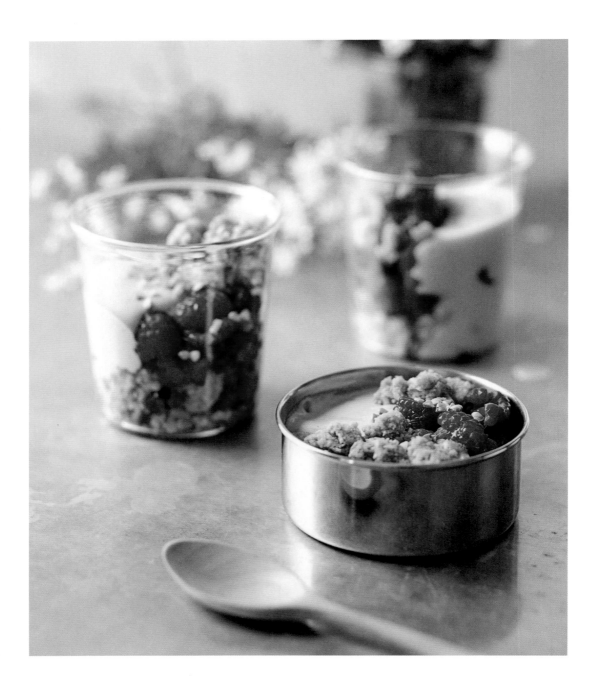

Raw Cashew Crumble with Cashew Cream

This crumble tastes like my memory of (naughtily) eating unbaked crumble dough as a kid (but this one won't give you a tummy ache!). It is thrown together in moments from store-cupboard staples and is great for making any bento a bit extra special. Pack it in a small leak-proof container to take with you. As with all of my sweets, it's more of a mini-meal/snack rather than a sugar bomb. If your blender jug is big you may need to double the amounts for the ingredients to blend properly. Instead of cashew cream, you can use any plant-based yogurt but I really recommend giving the cream a go, it's magic how it comes together 'just' from nuts!

Makes 2–3 portions.

Fridge life (crumble mix, minus fruit):
up to 2 weeks.
Freezer life (crumble mix, minus fruit):
up to 1 month.
Fridge life (cashew cream):
2–3 days.

Crumble

50g rolled jumbo oats
50g cashews
½ tsp vanilla powder
¼ tsp flaky sea salt
6–8 (40g) pitted dates, halved
2 tbsp odourless raw coconut oil
   (no need to melt)

Place the oats, cashews, vanilla and salt in a blender and blend to make a coarse flour. Add the dates (cutting them in half straight into the blender with scissors) and blend to a moist, coarse flour. Add the coconut oil and pulse a few times to form a crumble. Use straight from the blender jug. (Store leftovers in an airtight container in the fridge.)

Cashew Cream

60g cashews, quick-soaked for 10–15
   minutes or soaked overnight (see Tip)
4–6 (30g) pitted small dates, halved
   (soaked in a little hot water for
   10 minutes, if hard. Include the
   soaking water to blend)
¼ tsp vanilla powder
100ml water

Place all the cream ingredients in a blender and blend on the highest setting until very thick, light-coloured and fluffy – this will take 1 minute or so in a standard blender. If you prefer your cream a little thinner, add a little more water.

TO ASSEMBLE
Per Bento

100g frozen raspberries, or
   chopped up juicy fruit like
   ripe peaches

Layer the crumble mix, berries/ fruit and cashew custard either in small containers with lids to take away, or in glasses to eat at home.

TIP:
Quick-soak the cashews in plenty of hot water for 10–15 minutes, then drain and rinse cold under a tap, or soak them overnight, or at least 4 hours, in cold water, then drain.

Breakfast Granola Crumble

With your own granola (page 54), you can make a two-ingredient quick-crumble, which is great for breakfast or as a snack. If you don't have granola ready, make the instant version below. I like making these in portion sizes, either in glass or stainless steel food-prep containers (snap the lid on and take with you), silicon moulds as in the image or enamel dishes for eating at home. Or, make a larger crumble in a casserole and scoop portions into your bento as you go through the week. Tart, British apples are my favourites for crumble (when in season), maybe dressed up with a scatter of berries or stone fruit, but you can of course add anything you like. I remember an especially delicious one for friends while on holiday, using the fruit we had at hand – bananas, nectarines, pears and cherries with extra nuts and olive oil!

Makes 4 portions.
Fridge life: up to 5 days.

600g (5–6) apples, peeled if desired,
  cored and cut into small chunks

either use ready granola:
200g pre-prepped granola (page 54)
coconut palm sugar, to taste, optional
a drizzle of extra virgin olive oil, optional

or make instant granola:
100g rolled oats
1 tbsp sunflower seeds
1 tbsp flaxseeds
1 tbsp white (hulled) sesame seeds
2 tbsp nuts of your choice
2 tbsp brown rice syrup
1 tbsp extra virgin olive oil

plant-based yogurt, to serve, optional

TIP:
Delicious served with the
cashew cream on page 65.

Preheat the oven to 180°C/350°F/gas mark 4. Spread the chopped apples either in a casserole (about 25cm x 15cm), or four separate 1-portion baking trays (these can be metal bento boxes or glass or enamel storage containers, or silicon baking trays, like in the image).

If using pre-prepped granola, scatter a little sugar over the apples and top with granola. If using olive oil, drizzle it over the granola (this makes it crispier).

If making instant granola, add the granola ingredients to a bowl and combine well, then top the apples with the mixture.

Give the tray a little shake to combine the fruit and granola slightly. The total layer should be 4–5cm thick. Bake for 15–20 minutes, until the top is tanned and you can see fruit juices starting to bubble around the edges. Turn the oven off and leave the crumble in for a further 10 minutes, then remove (this makes the most of the oven heat). Let it cool completely, then cover and store in the fridge, or pack in a bento.

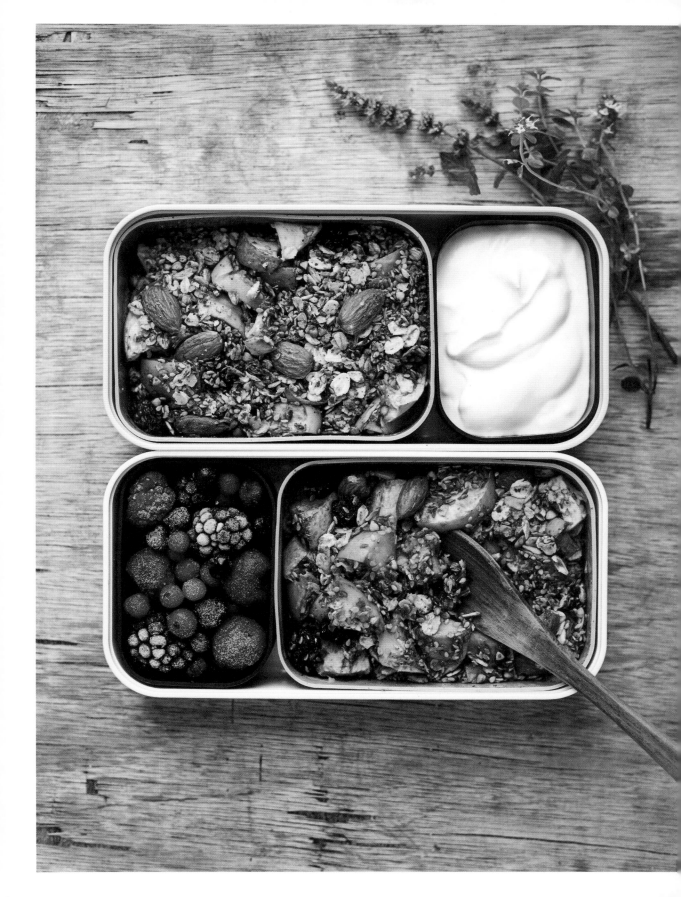

No-bake Matcha Brownies

Pretty little treats for your bento! Matcha green tea powder can be used in a similar way to cacao powder and, just like cacao, it adds both flavour (a subtle, multi-layered green flavour that I'm personally addicted to), and an uplifting effect. I use high-quality 'ceremonial-grade' matcha for this recipe. In Japan, matcha-flavoured white chocolate is an art form in itself, so I've played with it here to make a show-stopping coating (but you can roll your dough into small naked balls instead if you prefer!).

The recipe is easy to double, or triple, in a food processor (for one batch a reasonably strong blender will work well). The oats add creaminess and make the bites lighter, brown rice syrup adds a slight chewiness and miso rounds everything off beautifully.

Makes about 18 x 3cm square pieces.
Fridge life: up to 3 weeks.

Line a small baking tin
(a loaf tin, about 20 x 10cm, works well)
with baking paper.

Base
50g cashews
50g almonds (blanched if possible)
50g rolled jumbo oats
3 tbsp brown rice syrup
1 tbsp raw coconut oil (no need to melt it)
1 tbsp matcha powder
1 tsp brown rice miso paste

Coating
20–40g vegan white chocolate
  (iChoc is ideal)
½ tbsp raw coconut oil
½ tsp matcha powder

For the base, line a small baking tin (a loaf tin, about 20 x 10cm, works well) with baking paper. Place the nuts and oats in a blender or food processor and process to a coarse flour. Add all the remaining base ingredients and process until the mixture looks moist and just starts lumping together. Squish the mixture into the lined tin to form an even base.

For the coating, melt the white chocolate and coconut oil together. You can either do this in a small heatproof bowl placed over a pan of simmering water, or use a microwave. Spread half of it evenly over the base. Using a fork, whisk half the matcha powder into the remaining melted chocolate and drizzle half of it, or a little more, over the base in a random way.

Mix the remaining matcha and melted chocolate together for a dark green final touch and drizzle this over the base, again, the more random the better. Drag a cocktail stick through the white and green chocolates to create patterns.

Chill in the fridge to firm up, then cut into triangles or squares using a big, sharp knife. For the neatest results, heat the knife by dipping it in hot water and wipe it between cuts. Stack the brownies in an airtight container using a piece of baking paper between layers to keep the coating tidy-looking (optional!). Store in the fridge.

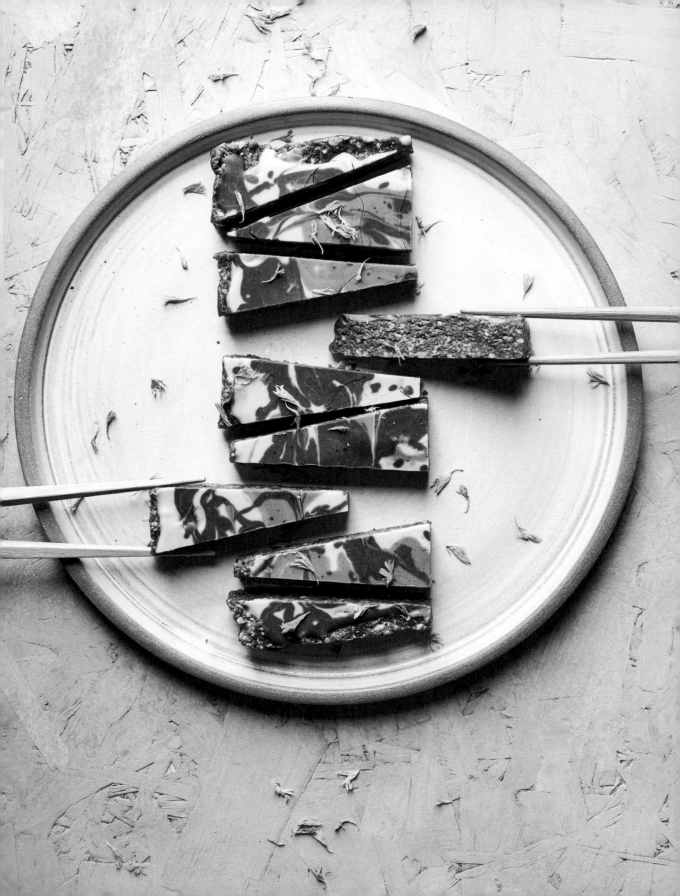

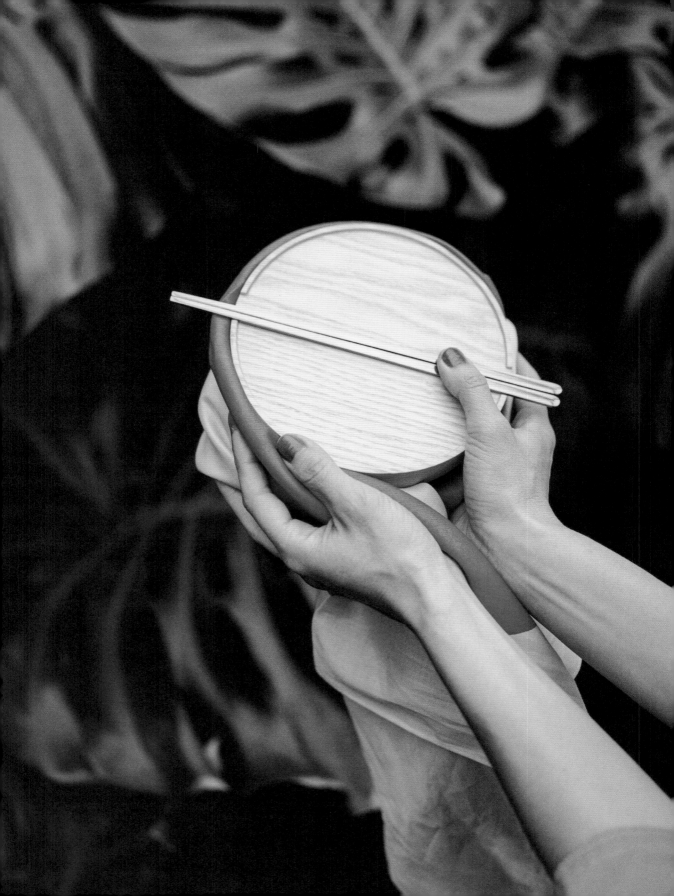

15-MINUTE BENTO

Bento in a hurry, full of flavour and power!
Since making bento almost daily, a few recipes
and tricks keep coming back again and again
because they simply work. Pack the most you can
– with the least time and effort!

Granola Salad Bento

The more crunchy toasted nuts and seeds you can get into this salad, the better! If your potion cabinet (pages 38–44) is stocked up, great, just pile your ready-toasted nuts and seeds in here, otherwise get your pan out and toast a few handfuls. I rarely pre-mix salad dressings for bento, but just drizzle everything over and hope that movement and time will merge everything by lunchtime (no one has complained yet!). You can leave the dressing out altogether, just add more nuts and seeds and a sprinkle of salt. You can use the little gem leaves whole, as edible spoons – great also if you make this as a big sharing dish.

Makes 1 bento.
Fridge life: 24 hours.

Granola Salad

2–3 sprouting broccoli stems, cut or
   pulled apart into bite-sized chunks
1 celery stick, thinly sliced
3–4 little gem lettuce leaves
1 portion of pre-prepped quinoa
   (page 31)
½ carrot, grated
1 overnight egg (page 51), peeled and
   quartered, optional

Start by quick-blanching the broccoli: place it in a heatproof bowl and pour boiling water over to submerge. Leave for 5 minutes, then drain in a strainer and cool completely under a cold running tap. While you're waiting for the broccoli, chop and grate your veggies.

For the toppings, toast the nuts and seeds, if you don't have any pre-prepped: heat a dry frying pan over a medium heat, add a few handfuls of almonds, sunflower and sesame seeds and stir occasionally until fragrant and a little tanned, 2–3 minutes. Tip onto a chopping board and chop roughly.

Dressing:
½ tbsp each olive oil and flaxseed oil
½ tbsp garlic-infused soy sauce (page 47)
½ tbsp clear honey or maple syrup
1 tsp balsamic vinegar
sea salt and freshly ground black pepper,
   to taste

Toppings:
3 tbsp savoury granola or saltwater-
   toasted nuts and seeds (pages 43–44)
   or freshly toasted almonds
   and sunflower seeds
1 tbsp toasted sesame seeds (page 41)
pink peppercorns, to taste
1 strawberry, sliced, optional

TO ASSEMBLE

Use a leak-proof box or big glass jar with a lid for this bento. Start with a layer of broccoli and celery, with the whole lettuce leaves placed at the edges, ready to use as edible scoops (if using a jar, leave the leaves to last). Add a layer of quinoa, then carrot and egg, if using. Drizzle all the dressing ingredients over and finish by piling on the nuts and seeds, and a few pink peppercorns (crushed between your fingers). Close your box, or jar, and pack in a bento bag or furoshiki with a fork.

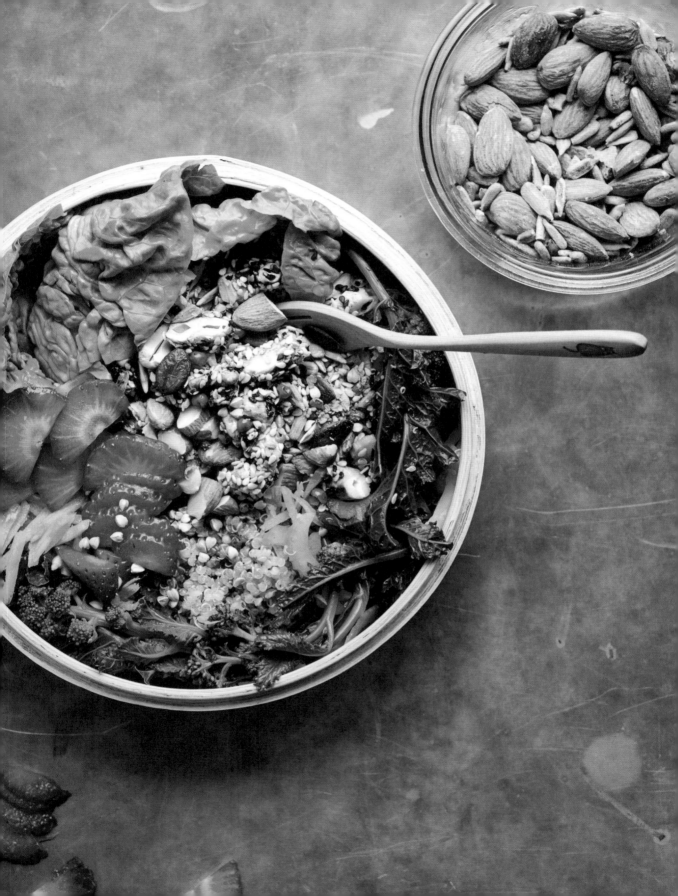

Lazy Tamago Bento

Making 'tamago-yaki' – Japanese rolled omelette – the traditional way may seem a little daunting, but here is my fail-proof, super-reduced version that's ready in 2 minutes (yes, really!). It was one of the first recipes Andy tested for this book and he makes it all the time now for his own bentos. Layering the egg with a nori sheet in the pan makes it easy to flip and fold, and adds both nutritional value and good looks. Lazy Tamago is great practise before attempting the original Tamago-yaki – Rolled Omelette Bento (see page 134).

Makes 1 bento.
Eat the same day.

Lazy Tamago

1 organic egg
a little oil, to fry
a pinch each of sea salt and chilli flakes
½ or 1 nori sheet

Crack your egg into a glass jar with a lid, add salt and chilli, close the lid tight and give it a really good shake.

Heat a medium frying pan over a medium heat until hot, then drizzle with a little oil. Pour the egg mixture into the pan and quickly tilt to cover the surface like a crepe. Immediately (yes!) place the whole nori sheet on top and within seconds you'll see your tamago curling up at the sides, ready to fold in three. Slide onto a clean chopping board and leave to cool slightly before cutting into bite-sized strips.

Variation:

Instead of salt in the mixture, use ½ tsp tamari.

TO ASSEMBLE

1 portion of pre-prepped quinoa-sunflower rice (page 35)
a few radicchio leaves, or any other salaf leaf
2cm cucumber, very thinly sliced (1–2mm), using a mandolin if you have one
tamari seeds (page 44) or any toasted nuts and seeds
½ tsp brown rice vinegar
pinch each of sea salt and gochugaru (Korean pepper)
1 wedge of (blood) orange
toasted sesame seeds (page 41), to taste
herbs, to garnish, optional

Arrange the rice in one end of your box and use a piece of radicchio leaf as a bowl for the lazy tamago. Use baking paper to make a small pocket each for the cucumber slices and toasted nuts (page 116) and drizzle the rice vinegar over the cucumber and sprinkle with a little salt and gochugaru. The cucumber will marinate slightly by lunchtime. Add the orange and finish with a sprinkle of sesame and herbs, if using. Close your box and pack in a bento bag or furoshiki with chopsticks or a fork.

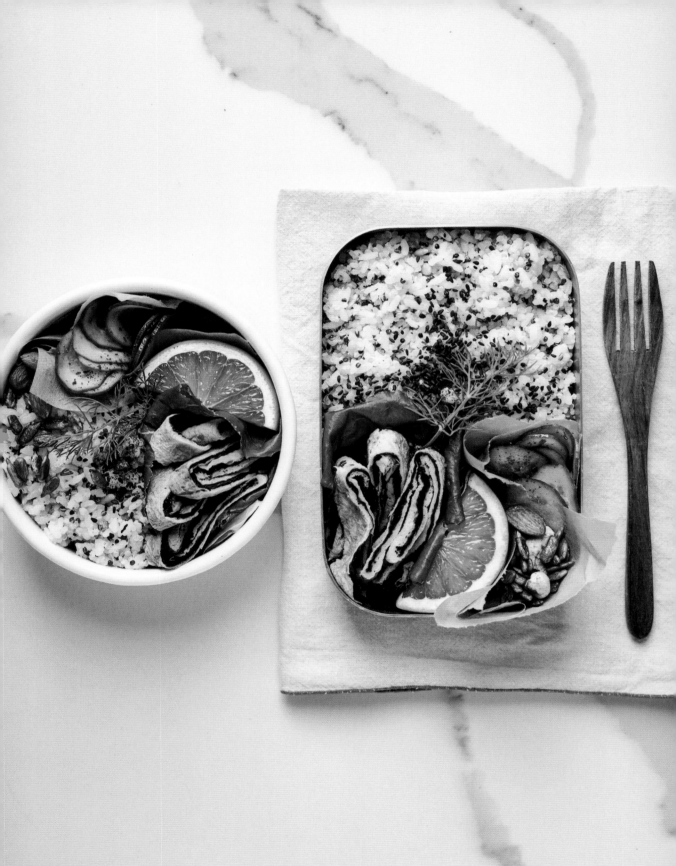

Busy Days Instant Noodle Bento

————

I ate soo many instant noodle meals as a university student – back then I had no idea I could make my own, wholesome version in minutes! Thin dry rice vermicelli rehydrates quickly in hot water, so just place them dry in a heatproof container, add a delicious miso paste and ginger soup base, plus raw veggies (you can use any veggie as long as it's sliced thin or grated). When you're ready to eat, it's just like the original – pour boiling hot water over, wait a few minutes and then slurp down your warm instant noodle soup.

Makes 1 portion.
Fridge life: up to 3 days as long as the noodles have not yet been rehydrated.

½ nest (50–75g) dry rice vermicelli
a handful of salad greens, like rocket, watercress or baby spinach
½ small carrot, grated
a small piece of red cabbage, cut into thin slices
1 tbsp brown rice miso paste
1 tbsp toasted sesame oil
1 tbsp tamari
2cm piece fresh ginger, washed but not peeled, finely grated straight into your bento
fresh chilli, sliced, or chilli flakes, to taste
fresh coriander, to taste, optional
a slice of lime, to serve, optional

Use a leak-proof box, or a repurposed jar with a lid for this bento. Break a whole, dry nest of noodles in half (over your sink, as pieces will fly everywhere!), then jam one half into your container together with the rest of the ingredients. No need to arrange neatly for this bento! Close tightly and pack your container in a bento bag or furoshiki with a fork or chopsticks.

To serve, remove the lime slice, if using, pour boiling water over to submerge the ingredients, close the lid, leave for 5 minutes or a little more, then open, squeeze the lime over and eat.

TIP:
Meal prep a few Busy Days Instant Noodle Bentos and keep ready to go in the fridge. Less perishable veggies like carrot, cabbage and broccoli are best used for this, salad greens and herbs can be added on the day.
   Cubed firm tofu or cooked beans are both great added to your bento as a protein boost.

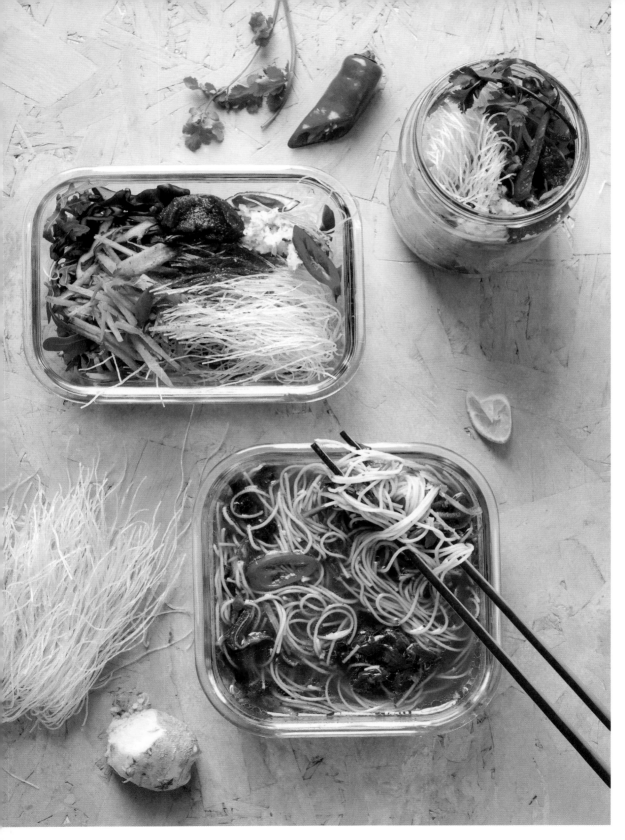

Hiya-yakko – Cool Tofu Scramble Bento

'Hiya-yakko' is a Japanese summer dish: a block of chilled silken tofu, perked up by soy sauce, grated fresh ginger and spring onions on top. I like making it into a bento, with colourful veggies and a sheet of nori inbetween the tofu/veggie topping and the rice base. Why the nori? By lunchtime, the tofu has released some liquid, which softens the nori which mixes with the other seasonings as you dig in – delicious!

Makes 1 bento.
Fridge life: up to 24 hours.

1 portion of pre-prepped 50/50 rice, or quinoa (pages 35 and 31)
½ nori sheet
a handful of salad greens, like rocket, watercress or baby spinach
¼ avocado, flesh scooped out or sliced
¼ pepper, thinly sliced
1 ripe tomato, roughly chopped
75–100g organic silken tofu
1cm piece fresh ginger, washed but unpeeled
1 tbsp tamari
1 spring onion, finely sliced
1 tbsp gomashio (any type) or toasted sesame seeds (pages 40–41)

Variation:

Instead of topping the tofu with tamari, ginger and spring onion on the tofu, try my Japanese friend Akki's topping: ½ tbsp toasted sesame oil, a good pinch of flaky sea salt and a small bunch of garlic chives, finely snipped with scissors.

TO ASSEMBLE

Use a leak-proof box. Make a bed of rice, as even as possible, and lay the nori on top. Rip bits off the nori to fit, and include all of it. Place the salad greens at one end of your bed and top it with the avocado, then place the pepper and tomato at the other end. If you have a square box you can make a diagonal shape, as in the image.

Drain the liquid from the tofu pack and gently slide out your preferred portion directly in between the two veggie mounds. You may need to push down on the tofu with a spoon or your clean hands to break it slightly. Finely grate the ginger over the tofu (using a microplane or box grater) then drizzle the tamari over and the spring onion too. Finish with the gomashio (or toasted sesame), in a small mound, to mix in when eating. Close your box and pack in a bento bag or furoshiki with a fork or chopsticks.

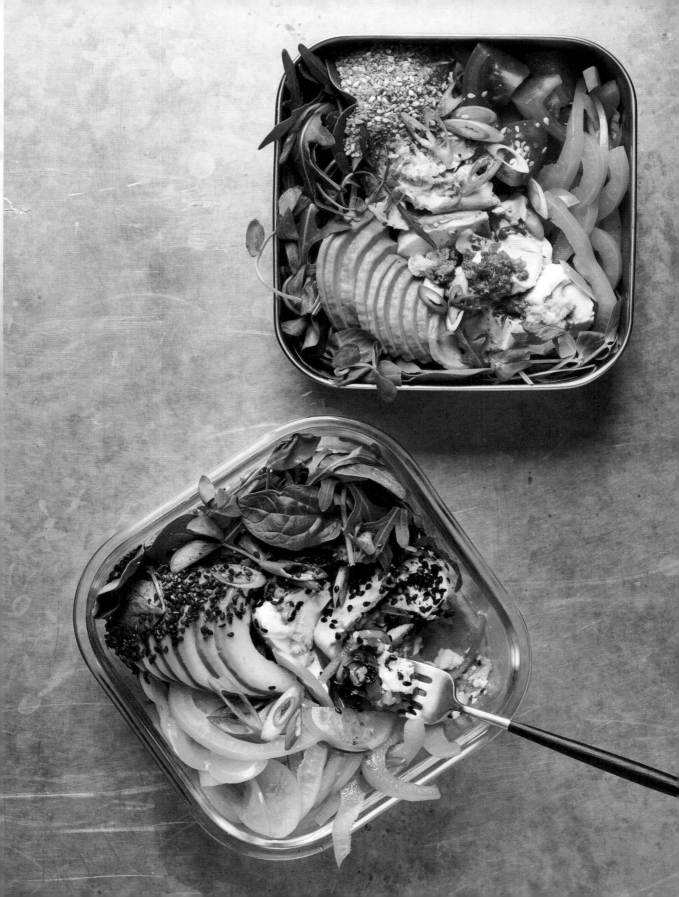

'Tack för Fisk-smörgåsen' Bento

It's rare I pack sandwiches to go, but when I eat at home I often have this 'Fisk smörgåsen' (fish sandwich) either on a good sourdough rye bread or corn or rye crackers. The name is the sentence Andy has memorised in Swedish (to thank my mum): 'Thanks for the fish sandwich'. Wild as these flavours may sound, it's one of my favourite flavour combinations: creamy avocado and omega-rich flaxseed oil, dulse seaweed and tangy sauerkraut. Fresh dulse is amazing but rare to find, so I use whole strands of dried dulse (not granules). You can use kalamata olives instead of dulse.

Makes 1 bento.
Eat the same day.

2 slices of (sourdough) rye bread
1 avocado
3g dried dulse seaweed, ripped in pieces
2 tbsp sauerkraut, juice drained off
½ tbsp flaxseed oil
flaky sea salt and freshly ground black
  pepper, to taste
a few chives, finely chopped or a few
  fronds of dill, torn
1 pear
a few radishes

Spread one slice of rye bread with half the avocado, top with the seaweed and sauerkraut and finish with a drizzle of flaxseed oil. Season with salt and pepper and fresh herbs, if using.

Spread the second slice of bread with the remaining avocado, close the sandwich and either pack as it is in a bento box, or wrap in baking paper. You may need to cut it to make it fit in your box. Add the pear and radishes to your box, or on the side. Pack your box or wrapped sandwich in a bento bag or furoshiki with a napkin.

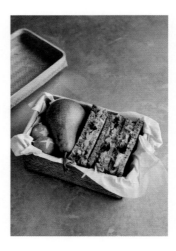

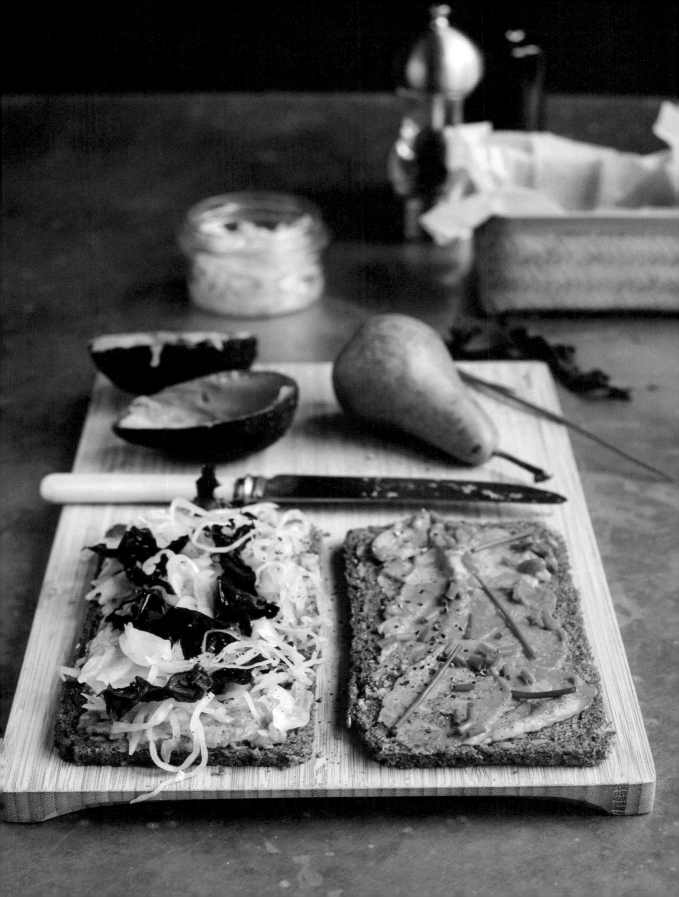

Thai Massaged Greens Bento

Everyone needs a little massage now and again, even your veggies!
Massaging is a way of gently 'cooking' or transforming vegetables without
applying heat. By adding salt and pressure (literally, massaging them), their
cellulose softens, their bulk reduces, they become easier to digest and there
are all kinds of interesting things you can do with their flavour and texture.
Experimenting with a raw food diet for a few years influenced my cooking a
lot, but eating exclusively raw foods is not something I'd do now (unless I lived
a very quiet, safe, non-materialistic life on a tropical mountain top…). Well,
until then I can always have this jar, and I'm definitely not complaining!

Makes 1 bento.
Fridge life: up to 2 days.

Thai massaged greens
makes 1–2 portions.
Fridge life: up to 3 days.

Thai Massaged Greens

1 pak choi, halved lengthways, then cut
into bite-sized chunks (see Tip)
50g (about 5cm small wedge) white
cabbage, finely sliced using a mandolin
if you have one
2 spring onions, finely sliced on the
diagonal (green part included)
1–2 red bird's eye chilli, cut into large
chunks on the diagonal
a little finely grated zest and the juice of
1 unwaxed lime
4cm piece fresh ginger, finely grated,
juice hand-squeezed straight into the
mix (pulp discarded)
2 tbsp umesu seasoning or 1 tsp sea salt
½ tbsp coconut palm sugar

While the noodles soak, chop your pak
choi, cabbage and spring onions and
place them in a sturdy plastic bag along
with the rest of the Thai massaged greens
ingredients. Remove all the air from the
bag and massage through the bag until
the vegetables are wilted and there is
a lot of liquid, about 1 minute. (Wash
the bag afterwards and reuse.) Store
leftovers in a glass jar with a lid in
the fridge.

TO ASSEMBLE

½ nest (50–75g) dry rice
vermicelli, rehydrated
(page 86)
½ mango, peeled and cut into
bite-sized chunks
50g firm, smoked tofu into bite-
sized chunks or 1 overnight
egg (page 51), peeled and
quartered
crispy coconut 'fakeon' or chilli-
toasted pumpkin seeds
(pages 43 and 44), to taste
a handful of salad greens

Use a leak-proof box or jar with
a lid. Tip the noodles in, then
the massaged greens including
its juice – this is your noodle
dressing. Top with the tofu or
egg. Finish with salad greens
and a scatter of 'fakeon' or
chilli-toasted pumpkin seeds (or
pack those in a separate, small
container to keep their crunch,
and add just before eating).
Close tightly and pack in a
bento bag or furoshiki with a
fork or chopsticks.

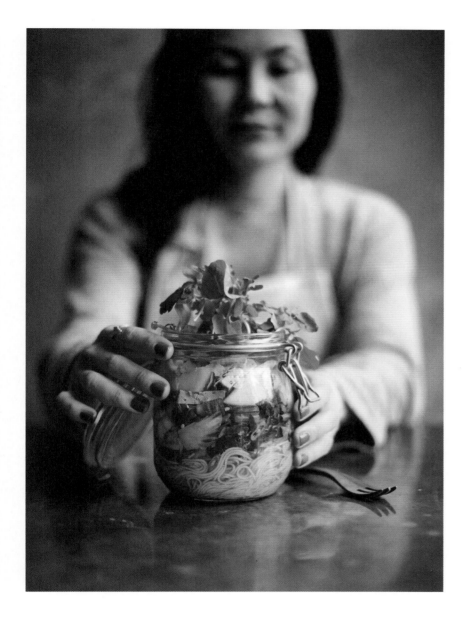

TIP:
Instead of pak choi you can use
4–5 leaves of kale (any type),
leaves ripped off its stalks and
torn into bite-sized chunks,
and stalks finely chopped and
added in, too.

Spicy Bamboo Garden Bento

Last summer I got obsessed with fermented, spicy jalapeño carrots made by my local producer and friends Pama Creations. I'd chop them up and mix with rice along with some of their liquid. This is my own quick-pickle version, with veggies arranged as a little garden! Quick-pickling and quick-blanching, both used in this bento (and many others, too), soften the edge of raw vegetables, gently 'raw cooking' them in minutes, with a minimum of fuss.

Makes 1 bento.
Eat on the same day.

Spicy quick-pickle carrots
makes 2 portions.
Fridge life: 1 week or more.

Spicy Quick-pickle Carrots

1 medium carrot (100g), peeled
½ tsp coconut palm sugar
½ tsp sea salt
1 tbsp brown rice vinegar
1–2 fresh jalapeño or other medium-hot chilli, thinly sliced, or 1 tsp chilli flakes

Cut the carrot in thin strips or discs, using a julienne slicer or mandolin if you have one, and place it with the pickling ingredients and chilli in a sturdy plastic bag. (It is better to use a bag rather than a bowl for this recipe, as you may not want to touch the fresh chilli with your bare hands.) Remove all the air and massage together through the bag until juicy and softened, a minute or more (wash and reuse the bag afterwards). Transfer to a glass storage container with a lid and store in the fridge.

Quick-blanched Veggies

2 small broccoli florets, cut into bite-sized pieces
3 asparagus spears, trimmed and cut into 5cm pieces

Place both the broccoli and asparagus in a heatproof bowl and pour boiling water over to submerge. Leave for 5 minutes, then drain in a strainer and cool completely under a cold running tap.

TO ASSEMBLE

1 portion of pre-prepped 50/50 Rice (page 35)
a handful of salad leaves
2 cherry tomatoes
¼ nectarine, cut into thin wedges
1 overnight egg (page 51), peeled and pixelated, or 2 tbsp cooked cannellini beans
lazy ra-yu chilli oil (page 48) or your favourite hot chilli sauce
a pinch of sea salt
cashew nut clusters (page 43), or any toasted nuts, to taste

Finely chop (if you like) half your quick-pickle and mix with the rice, along with half of the pickling juice. Arrange the rice in one side of your bento box (or shape the rice into an onigiri, page 114), and make a bed of salad leaves in the remaining space. Build your bamboo garden on top, bunching the asparagus together like bamboo trunks, broccoli as moss and fruit like rocks! Wedge the egg, or beans, in there somewhere too and top them with the oil, or chilli sauce, and salt. Finish with nuts (more rocks). Close your box and pack in a bento bag or furoshiki with a fork or chopsticks.

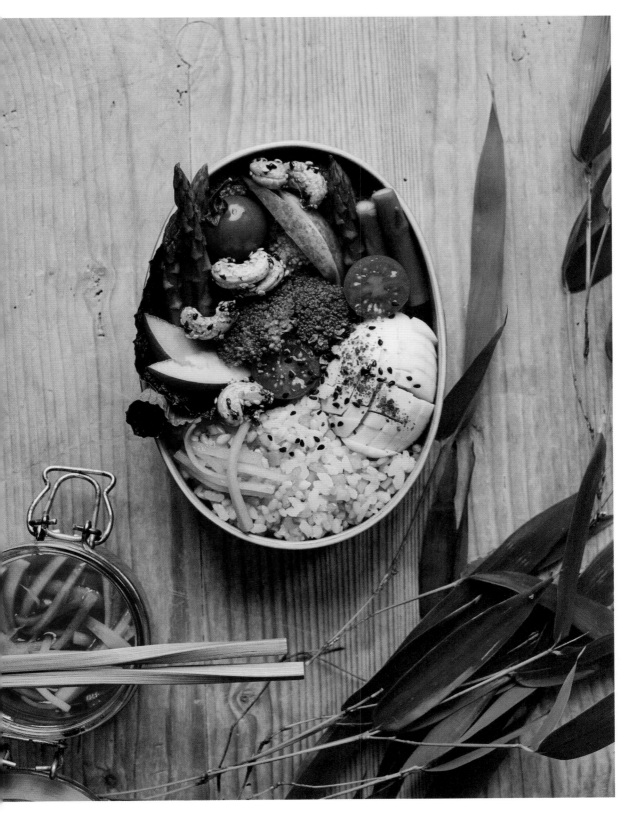

15-Minute Bento

No-wrap Summer Roll Bento

Who else loves Vietnamese rice paper rolls? They're my favourite, but a little too time-consuming for an everyday dish. With this bento, I get all their flavours in, without any of the wrapping! This works well as a big party salad too. The must-have ingredients are mint, cucumber, fresh chilli and peanuts – and if you haven't already tried adding watermelon to savoury salads this is the time. Pure summer magic!

Makes 1 bento.
Fridge life: 24 hours.

Rehydrating Rice Vermicelli

½ nest (50–75g) dry rice vermicelli

Break a whole, dry noodle nest in half (over your sink or a big bowl, as pieces will fly everywhere!), then place one half in a large, heatproof bowl and pour boiling water over to submerge. Weigh the noodles down with a lid or plate, if possible. Leave for 5 minutes, then drain in a strainer and cool completely under a cold running tap. Either let the noodles drip-dry in the strainer for 5 minutes or instantly spin them dry in a sturdy salad spinner. Depending on appetite you may want to rehydrate a little more vermicelli, up to 1 nest per bento, and add a little more seasoning/dressing to the recipe.

> TIP:
>
> Dry-toast the peanuts for a couple of minutes in a hot frying pan, then crush them against a chopping board using the base of a clean, big glass jar (or use a mortar and pestle).

Summer Roll Salad

2cm thin slice of watermelon, peeled and cut into bite-sized chunks
50g firm smoked tofu, cut into thin strips (Viana 'Real Smoked Tofu' is ideal)
3 tbsp raw peanuts, dry-toasted, and chopped or crushed (see Tip)
1 spring onion, finely chopped
fresh bird's eye chilli, sliced, to taste
a handful of salad greens, like rocket, watercress or baby spinach
¼ cucumber, peeled
1 small carrot
a small handful of fresh mint, torn
1 tbsp fish sauce (vegetarian) or 1 tbsp tamari
1 tbsp toasted sesame oil

While you wait for the noodles to rehydrate, cut your watermelon and tofu, toast the peanuts and chop the spring onion and chilli.

You'll need a big bento box for this bento. Layer the noodles and greens in your box.

Use a potato peeler to peel long strands of cucumber, then carrot, straight into the box (peeling firmly, away from your body, and rotating the vegetable after each peel may be the easiest). You will end up with a thin core of cucumber and carrot, cut these into rounds (check one o'clock in the image) and add them to the box too. Add the watermelon and tofu, then finish with the peanuts, spring onion, chilli and mint.

Add the fish sauce, oil and more chilli to a small leak-proof pot with a lid, to take with you as a dressing and pour over before eating. Close your box and pack in a bento bag or furoshiki with a fork or chopsticks.

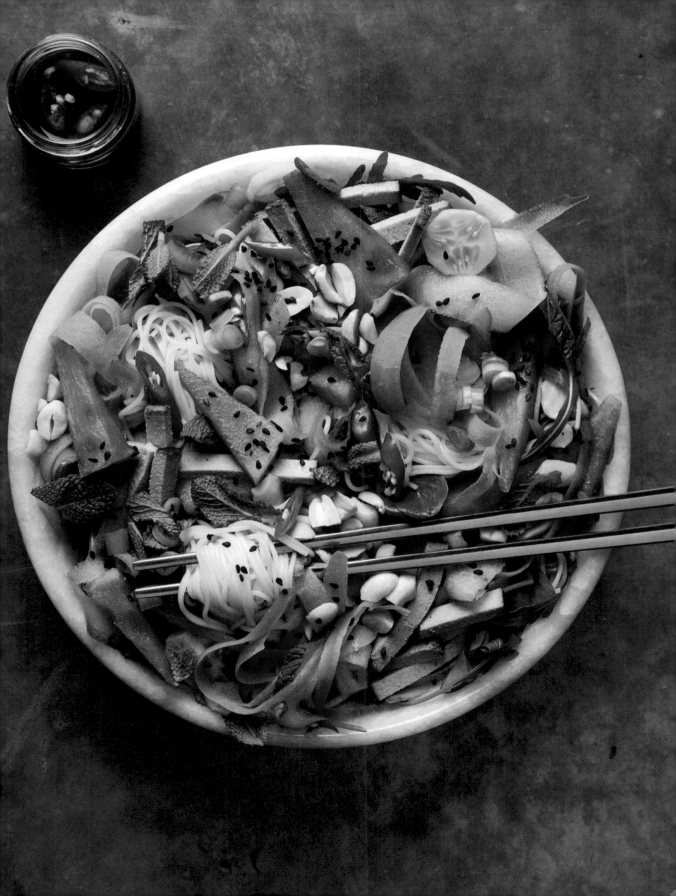

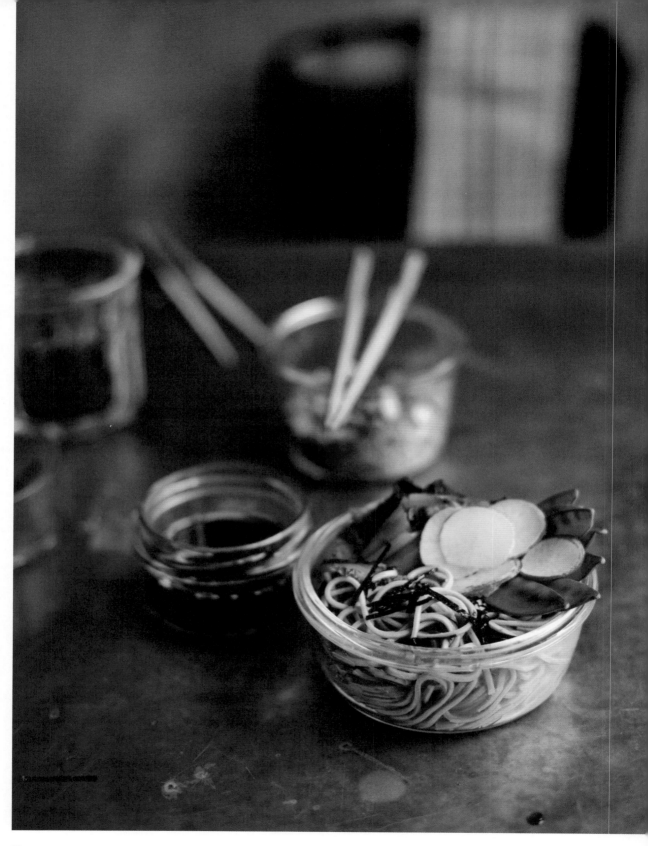

Lazy Zaru Soba Bento

If you've travelled in Japan in summer you may have tried 'zaru soba': chilled noodles dipped bite by bite in a refreshing seasoning broth. Since these noodles are eaten cold, they're perfect to put in a bento! To make 'proper' seasoning broth you need both time and bonito tuna flakes, which are delicious but can be hard to source, (and frankly, let's leave the last tuna we have left in the sea!). So here's my lazy version. I've used a touch of (vegetarian) fish sauce and wasabi, but you can leave both out and still have fabulous lazy zaru soba.

Makes 1 bento.
Fridge life: up to 2 days.

Soba Noodles

1 portion (85g) dry soba noodles
1 pak choi, halved lengthways
a handful of mangetout, trimmed, optional

Cook the soba according to the packet's instructions, adding the pak choi and mangetout, if using, to the water for the last 2 minutes of cooking time. Drain the soba and greens in a strainer then cool completely under a cold running tap. Either let them drip-dry in the strainer for 5 minutes or instantly spin them dry in a sturdy salad spinner.

TIP:

Chopsticks really are best for eating this bento! Mix the wasabi (if using) into the broth. Grab the broth with one hand, chopsticks in the other and dip the noodles in the broth, one mouthful at a time. If the noodles seem a little dry, moisten them by pouring a little broth over. The veggies are great dipped in the broth too.

Lazy Seasoning Broth

½ tbsp tamari
3 tbsp water
½ tsp maple syrup or agave syrup
⅛ tsp fish sauce (vegetarian), optional

Whisk together the broth ingredients in a leak-proof container with a lid that you will also use to transport it in. The container needs to be big enough for a chopstick-full of noodles!

TO ASSEMBLE

⅛ nori sheet, ripped or shredded with scissors (see nori confetti on page 38)
1 spring onion, finely sliced, optional
2–3 radishes, halved or cut into thin rounds
¼ avocado, flesh scooped out or sliced
seasoned nuts and seeds, any type (pages 43–44), to taste
1 portion wasabi from powder (page 49), to taste, optional

Pick out the pak choi halves and mangetout from the noodles and cut them into bite-sized chunks. Place the soba in your box and scatter with nori and spring onion, if using, then push the noodles to one side, and arrange the radish, avocado and nuts in the remaining space, in separate sections if possible. If you are using wasabi, shape it into a blob and place anywhere on the side of your soba. Close your box and pack in a bento bag or furoshiki with chopsticks and a napkin.

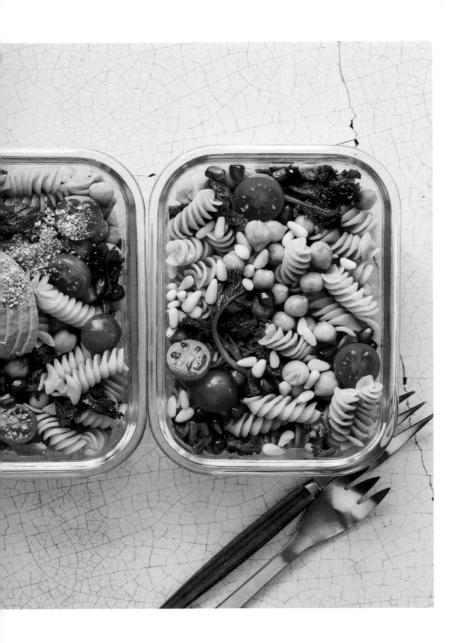

Pasta Surprise Bento

It's a standing joke between me and Andy that when he cooks dinner, four times out of five it will be a 'pasta surprise'. Well, the good thing about it is how easy and quickly it comes together – and we've started adding veggies to the cooking water for colour and added nutrients. Pasta surprise works well in a bento, just make sure you choose a pasta that will be delicious even when cold (I love Le Veneziane gluten-free spirals) and undercook it slightly. What to put inside can be your own surprise, but here is one simple red and green suggestion.

Makes 2–3 portions.
Fridge life: up to 2 days.

200g pasta, shells or spirals are great
½ head of broccoli, florets separated and cut, or torn, in halves
4–5 kale leaves, any type
240g cooked chickpeas (drained and rinsed, if using canned)

Dressing:
2 tbsp tamari sauce
1 tbsp extra virgin olive oil or flaxseed oil
1 tbsp balsamic vinegar

Toppings:
2 tbsp red gomashio (page 41), and/or a handful of pine nuts
½ avocado, flesh scooped out or sliced
a few cherry tomatoes and/or a handful of pomegranate seeds, optional

Cook the pasta according to the packet's instructions. While it cooks, prepare the broccoli and rip the kale leaves off their stems, then finely chop the stems.

Two minutes before the pasta is done (remember to undercook it slightly), add the vegetables and chickpeas to the cooking water, bring to the boil again and continue cooking for the remaining time. Drain in a strainer and cool completely under a cold running tap. Drip-dry in the strainer for 5 minutes or instantly spin dry in a sturdy salad spinner.

Return to the pan (best if the pan has also been cooled under the tap together with the pasta) and add all the dressing ingredients. Stir or shake the pan to combine. Tip into bento boxes and add the toppings. Close your box and pack in a bento bag or furoshiki with a fork or chopsticks.

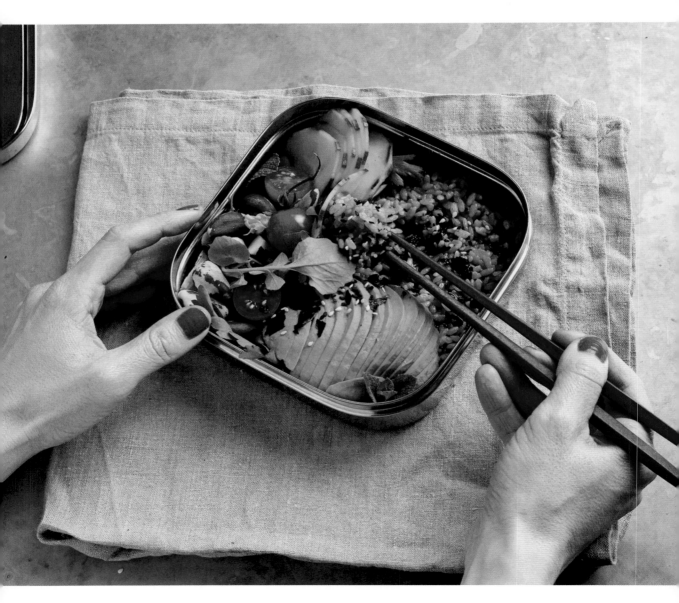

BENTO POWER

Smashed Nori Roll Bento

I love a classic sushi nori roll! What about skipping a step (or two), but using all of its flavours, with a basic sushi technique, and have a non-rolled roll within minutes? By adding warm rice to a seasoning liquid and letting it cool down while gently folding, we get that slightly chewy sushi-rice texture and the dipping sauce (soy) has been added to the rice already! Either use freshly cooked rice (this is when a rice cooker comes in really handy) or heat up leftovers (See Tip). Dijon mustard gives a very similar pungency to wasabi.

Makes 1 bento.
Fridge life: 24 hours.

TIP:
To heat rice microwave-free, use an ordinary steamer basket, lined with a little baking paper to stop the rice from falling through. Steam for 5 minutes, until piping hot.

Smashed Nori Roll

2 tsp coconut palm sugar or
  1 tsp agave syrup
2 tsp tamari
1 tsp brown rice vinegar
1 tsp dijon mustard
1 tsp black toasted sesame seeds
  (page 41)
200–250g warm, cooked white Japanese
  rice (about ½ batch), page 29
1 nori sheet, torn into small pieces, plus
  some reserved to finish

Use your bento box as a mixing bowl, stirring the sugar, tamari, vinegar, mustard and sesame together, then add the warm rice and nori and combine with a spoon, without crushing the grains too much, until the rice has cooled enough to add the raw veggies (without wilting them), about a minute.

TO ASSEMBLE

1 avocado, flesh scooped out
  or sliced
a handful of salad greens
10cm piece of cucumber, thinly
  sliced (use a mandolin if you
  have one)
a small handful of Brazil nuts
a couple of cherry tomatoes,
  halved
1 overnight egg (page 51),
  optional
toasted sesame seeds (page 41),
  to sprinkle

Push the rice to one side of the box and top it with avocado. Line the rest of the space with salad greens and top it with cucumber, nuts, tomato and egg, if using. Finish with a sprinkle of sesame. Close your box and pack in a bento bag or furoshiki with a fork or chopsticks.

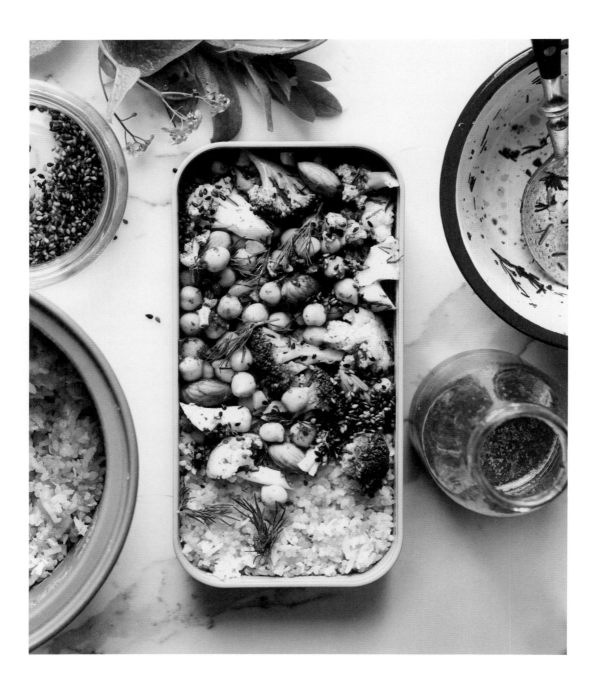

Baltic Sea Samurai Bento

The fresh dill and sweet-sour marinade with a touch of seaweed is the Baltic Sea Samurai here. I like to think of this as 'stove-free cooking' – letting ingredients (raw vegetables and active seasonings) slowly transform overnight. If you prepare this in the morning, there should still be enough time for the ingredients to marinate by lunchtime. I've soaked the almonds in water overnight, which makes them puff up, get softer, creamier tasting and filling in a whole new way.

Makes 1 bento.
Fridge life: up to 2 days.

2 tbsp whole almonds
2 small cauliflower florets (about 50g)
2 small broccoli florets (about 50g)
1 tsp apple cider vinegar
2 tsp coconut palm sugar
1 tsp aonori seaweed or ¼ sheet nori, finely crumbled
a couple of dill sprigs, torn, plus extra to garnish
½ tsp sea salt, smoked if possible
freshly ground pepper, to taste
50g cooked chickpeas (drained and rinsed, if using canned)

If you are preparing this in the evening, place the almonds in a small bowl, cover in cold water and leave to soak overnight. Cut the cauliflower and broccoli into small pieces including stalk. Add vinegar, sugar, seaweed, dill, salt and pepper to a mixing bowl, then add the veggies and chickpeas and combine. Place a second bowl on top of the salad mixture and weigh it down with something heavy (e.g. a can of food). In the morning, drain the almonds and add them to the salad.

If you are preparing this in the morning, follow the instructions as above, but mix the almonds into the salad right away, just as they are.

TO ASSEMBLE

1 pre-prepped grainy Japanese rice (page 34), or quinoa (31)
1 tbsp tamari seeds or chilli toasted pumpkin seeds (page 44)
1 tablespoon Korean-style dressing (page 47), optional

Pack the grains in one end of your bento box and fill the rest with salad, pouring the marinating liquid over the grains as a dressing. Drizzle over a little Korean-style dressing, if you like. Garnish with extra dill and tamari seeds. Close your box and pack in a bento bag, or furoshiki, with a fork or chopsticks.

Seoul Stand-up Noodle Bento

Here's a refreshing summer bento – or a jar, if you like. There's something satisfying about seeing these colour-popping layers build up! The Korean-style dressing is a killer and easy to shake together in a minute. If you like to make your Stand-up a little more substantial, add some avocado, cubed firm tofu or an overnight egg (page 51).

Makes 1 bento.
Fridge life: up to 24 hours.

½ nest (50–75g) dry rice vermicelli
a handful of frozen peas, straight
  from the freezer
½ tbsp instant dried wakame seaweed
2 tbsp Korean-style dressing (page 47)
a few peeled segments of red grapefruit
  or pomelo
¼ cucumber, thinly sliced (use a mandolin
  if you have one)
a handful of salad leaves, torn
saltwater-toasted nuts and seeds (page
  44) or toasted almonds and sunflower
  seeds, to taste

Start by rehydrating the rice vermicelli, see page 86, adding the frozen peas and wakame along with the dry noodles to soak in the hot water.

Use a leak-proof box, or jar with a lid. Tip the noodle mix in, drizzle the dressing over, then either gently shake the box/jar to mix together or use chopsticks to stir. Add the citrus segments, cucumber and as much salad as you can squeeze in before closing the lid. Add the seasoned nuts and seeds to a separate jar and either eat as they are or sprinkle over the noodles at lunchtime. Pack everything in a bento bag or furoshiki with a fork or chopsticks.

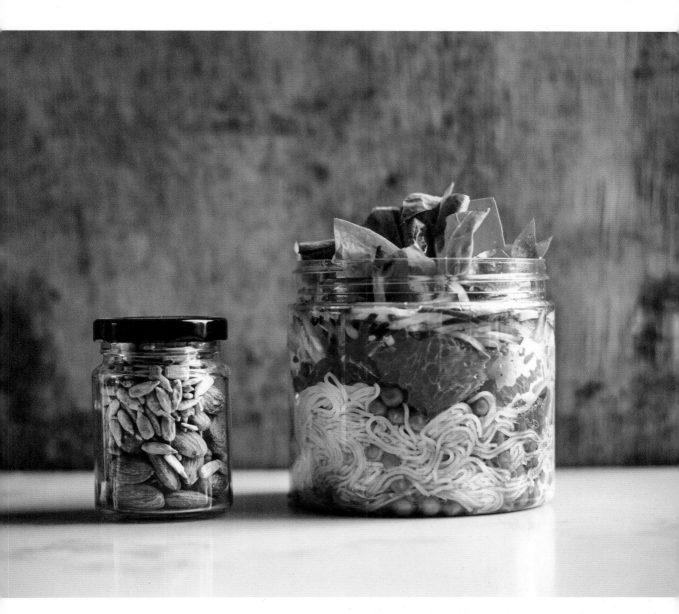

15-Minute Bento

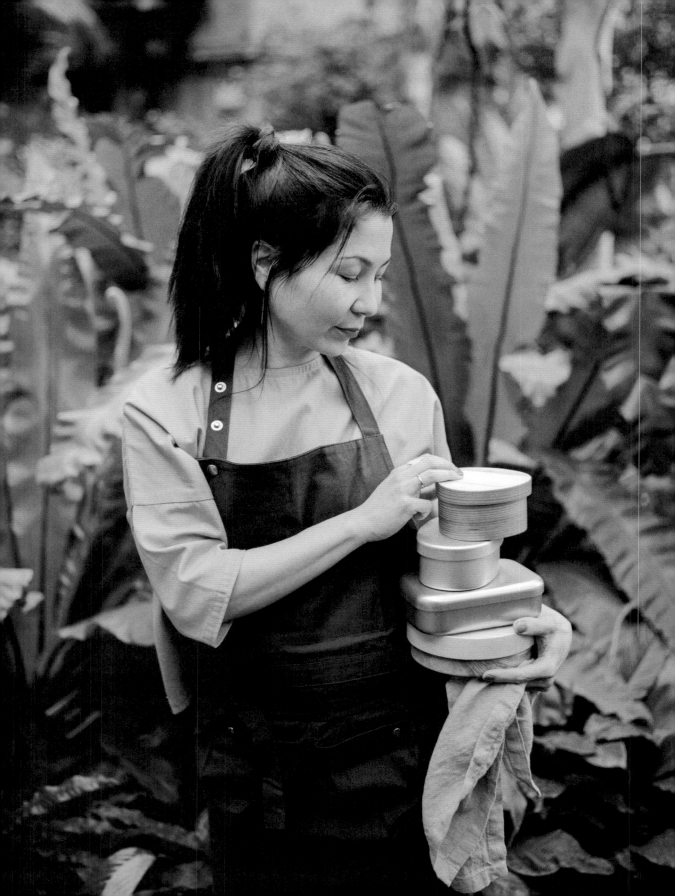

EVERYDAY BENTO

365 Bento power. My most-used, most versatile recipes, for bento but also for any time of day and occasion. Bento is modular by nature and these recipes are too – either make the full recipe, or pick and mix to make your own bento favourite!

Variety of Bento
(and Pulled King Oyster Mushrooms and Smoky Maple-roasted Beets)

I will admit, this is the bento meal-prep of my dreams! I've pulled together some of my absolute favourites here, all of which can be made ahead and keep well. In reality, even a couple of these dishes, along with a pot or two of rice, some fresh produce, tofu (pictured) or overnight eggs will set you up for a week of great bento! Overleaf I show how they can be used over a few days to make a variety of bento. Pulled mushrooms? However much I wish, I didn't come up with this amazing technique, all credit goes to my friend Derek Sarno of Wicked Healthy (and his literally magic ways with shrooms). It's a must-try.

Makes 4–5 bento.
Fridge life for all the dishes:
up to 5 days.

Pulled King Oyster (Eryngii) Mushrooms

4 king oyster (eryngii) mushrooms, trimmed (see Tip)
2 tbsp extra virgin olive oil
2 tbsp tamari
pinch of mild dried chilli flakes or chilli powder (I like ancho or chipotle chilli, but you can use any)

Preheat the oven to 190°C/375°F/ gas mark 5, and line a baking tray with baking paper.

Pull the mushrooms by using a fork and 'combing' the stalks lengthways into shreds on a chopping board. Include the caps too, torn into pieces. Using your hands, combine the mushroom shreds and caps with the seasonings on the lined tray, then spread out thinly.

Roast in the oven until most of the liquid has gone, 30 minutes, stirring once halfway through. Remove from the oven and leave to cool before packing in your bento box and storage container (store leftovers in the fridge).

TIP:
If you can't find king oyster mushrooms (pictured), make a batch of either the rawmari mushrooms (page 118) or a double batch of the umami bomb mix (page 129).

Smoky Maple-roasted Beets

1kg beetroots (mixed colours if possible), scrubbed and cut into bite-sized chunks (see Tip)
1 tbsp extra virgin olive oil
pinch of sea salt
1 tbsp maple syrup
1 tbsp tamari
½ tbsp apple cider vinegar
1 tsp smoked paprika

Preheat the oven to 200°C/400°F/ gas mark 6, and line a baking tray with baking paper (see Tip).

Pile the beetroot, olive oil and salt on the lined tray and combine, coating all the beetroot chunks in oil. (To save your hands from going red, you can grab the edges of the paper and gently shake the beetroot inside.)

Roast on the highest shelf in the oven until the chunks are slightly charred at the edges, 20–30 minutes. Turn the oven off and leave the beetroot to finish cooking in the residual heat for 10 minutes.

Mix the maple syrup, tamari, vinegar and smoked paprika in a large mixing bowl. Add the hot beetroot chunks and toss to combine. Cover with a plate and leave to marinate overnight. The next day, pack in your bento box and storage container (store leftovers in the fridge).

Pak Choi Quick-pickle

2 pak choi, quartered lengthways
2 tbsp tamari or fish sauce (vegetarian)
the juice and a little finely grated zest of 1 unwaxed lime or lemon
½ tsp sea salt
red bird's eye chilli, cut into chunks on the diagonal, or chilli flakes, to taste
4cm piece fresh ginger, peeled and cut into thin strips

Crush the pak choi firmly against your chopping board with the heel of your hand – cracking it makes it soak up the marinade better. Place in a bowl and add the rest of the ingredients, combining well.

The pickle is ready to pack in your bento box straight away, but is best after it has been left to marinate overnight. To do this, place a second, clean bowl on top of the pickle mix with a weight inside (e.g. a can of food) and leave in the fridge overnight. Before using in your bento, cut the pak choi into bite-sized chunks (store leftovers in the fridge).

TIP:
You can use a mix of beetroot and carrots, or all carrots, if you prefer. As soon as the pulled mushrooms are out of the oven, turn the temperature up (as shown) and roast the beetroot mix straight after.

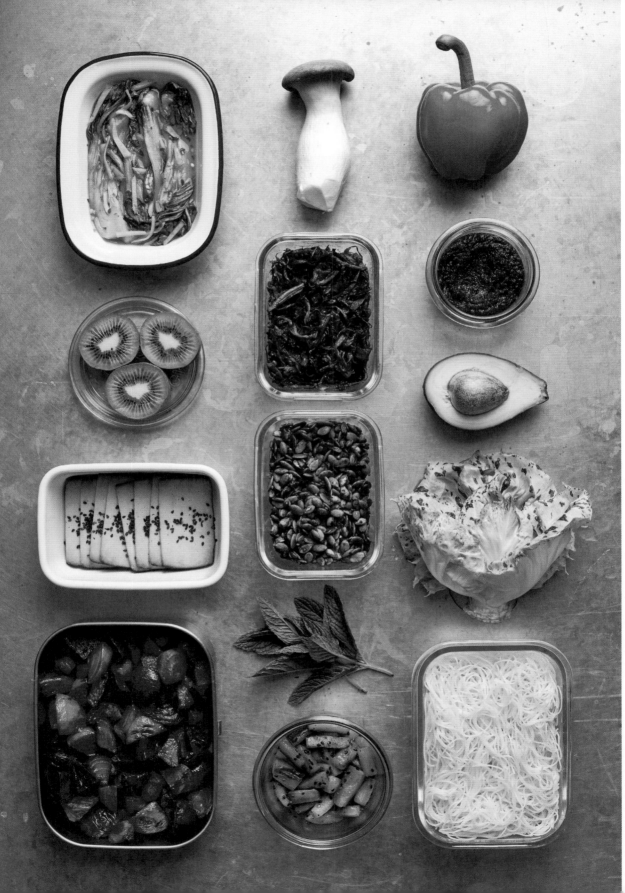

Cheatin' Gochujang Sauce

Prepare one batch, page 48.

Chilli-toasted Pumpkin Seeds

Prepare one batch, page 44.

Korean Cucumber

1 cucumber, peeled
1 tsp sea salt
4cm piece fresh ginger, washed but not
  peeled, finely grated
1 tsp toasted sesame oil
1 tsp gochugaru (Korean red pepper)
  or a pinch of chilli flakes
2 tsp black toasted sesame seeds
  (page 41), optional

Halve the cucumber lengthways and
remove the seeds with a small spoon.
Halve each half again lengthways and
then again (you'll end up with 8 long
pieces). Cut into 3–4cm chunks and
place in a large bowl.

Sprinkle the cucumber with salt and
soften it by massaging the chunks with
your hands, in the bowl, squeezing the
pieces hard enough for them to soften,
start looking slightly translucent and
release liquid. Rinse off the salt in a
strainer, then pat them dry in a clean
tea towel.

Place the chunks in a glass jar with a
lid and squeeze the grated ginger over
(discard the pulp), then add all the
remaining ingredients and shake well to
combine. Pack in your bento box and
store leftovers in the fridge.

> *TIP:*
> Instead of the seasonings
> above, you can use 1 tbsp of
> the gochujang sauce you have
> prepared and mix thoroughly with
> the softened cucumber chunks.

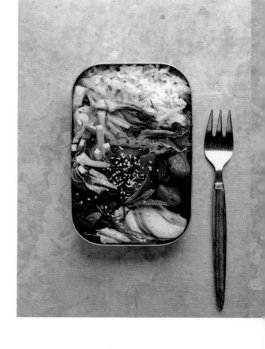

TO ASSEMBLE

> *TIP:*
> For all the quick-pickle recipes
> in this book, use the marinating
> liquid (as well as the pickled
> veggie) when packing your
> bento as it's full of flavour and
> nutrients. Pour the liquid over
> the rice, noodles or salad
> veggies to season them.

Bento 1: with Rice

1 portion pre-prepped rice (any from the
  Base Recipes –pages 28–37)
about ¼ batch each of the:
  smoky maple-roasted beets
  pak choi quick-pickle
  pulled king oyster mushrooms
50g firm, smoked tofu
¼ avocado, sliced
toasted sesame seeds (page 41),
  to garnish

Arrange the rice in one end of your
box. Cut the pak choi into bite-sized
chunks and place on top of the rice,
drizzle some of its marinating juice
over the rice, too. In the remaining
space, add the beets, mushrooms, tofu
and avocado, all separated by salad
leaves. Finish with a sprinkle of sesame.

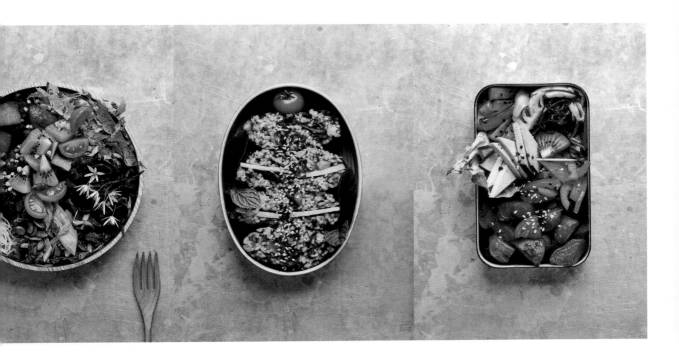

Bento 2: with Noodles

1 portion rehydrated rice vermicelli
   (page 86)
1 tbsp cheatin' gochujang sauce
a few salad leaves, shredded
about ¼ batch each of the:
   smoky maple-roasted beets
   pak choi quick-pickle
   pulled king oyster mushrooms
chilli-toasted pumpkin seeds, to taste
1 cherry tomato, quartered
½ kiwi, peeled and sliced or flesh
   scooped out
a sprinkle of buckwheat, optional
wild garlic flowers, optional

Arrange the rice noodles at one end
of your box and dollop the gochujang
sauce on top. Line the remaining space
with salad leaves and top with the
beets, pak choi, mushrooms, pumpkin
seeds, tomato and kiwi. Finish with a
sprinkle of buckwheat and wild garlic
flowers, if using.

Bento 3: Onigirazu

300g pre-prepped rice (any from the
   Base Recipes – pages 28–37)
1 tbsp cheatin' gochujang sauce
about ¼ batch each of the:
   Korean cucumber, chopped
   pulled king oyster mushrooms
2 nori sheets
50g firm, smoked tofu, in thin slices like in
   the image on the previous spread
toasted sesame seeds (page 41),
   to garnish
a few fresh mint leaves, to garnish,
   optional

Mix the rice with the gochujang sauce,
cucumber and mushrooms. Make
2 onigirazu (sushi sandwiches),
following the instructions on pages
130–131, loading the tofu slice in
the middle.

Bento 4: Grain-free

about ¼ batch each of the:
   smoky maple-roasted beets
   pak choi quick-pickle
   Korean cucumber
   pulled king oyster mushrooms
a few salad leaves, shredded
50g firm, smoked tofu
¼ red pepper, sliced
½ kiwi, peeled and sliced or flesh
   scooped out
toasted sesame seeds (page 41),

Arrange the beets in one end of your
box and line the rest of the space with
salad leaves, keeping some to use as
separators for the pak choi pickle (cut
into bite-sized pieces), cucumber and
mushrooms. Cut the tofu into slices as
shown in the image (or as you wish)
and spear them with a cocktail stick, to
look cute and be fun to eat! Finish with
the red pepper and kiwi and a sprinkle
of sesame.

Green Theme Bento

This is one of my bento classics, from when I was just getting in to the swing of making and Instagramming them. If you have a rice cooker, then this is one of the easiest types of bento to make, just load your cooker at night to have rice ready in the morning, when you quickly fry your egg and pack your veggies (that are simply cut and placed in the box with seasonings drizzled over). Plain rice always tastes great with nori, (black) sesame and salt!

Makes 1 bento.
Fridge life: 24 hours.

Sesame-fried Egg

a little toasted sesame oil, to fry
1 tsp sesame seeds (any type, not toasted)
1 organic egg
a pinch of sea salt

Heat a frying pan over a medium heat. Add a little oil and scatter half of the sesame seeds into the oil to fizzle for a few seconds, then crack the egg on top. Scatter the rest of the seeds, and salt, over the egg. For speed you can pop the yolk (avoid runny eggs, for bento food safety). When the yolk seems firm, flip and fry for a few more moments then slide onto a chopping board and cut into bite-sized strips (easier to pick out of the box) and leave to cool.

Green Theme Salad

50g savoy cabbage, saving 1 leaf to
  use as a separator in your bento
¼ green pepper, finely sliced
½ kiwi, peeled and sliced or
  flesh scooped out
1 tsp toasted sesame oil
½ tsp brown rice vinegar
a pinch of sea salt

Finely shred the cabbage and pepper and place straight into your bento box. Add the kiwi and drizzle over the sesame oil, vinegar and salt – no need to mix them before.

TO ASSEMBLE

1 portion of pre-prepped
  50/50 Rice (page 35)
2 tsp toasted sesame seeds,
  black (page 41)
a good pinch of sea salt
¼ nori sheet, cut or ripped into
  confetti (page 38)
25g soft-medium tofu, cubed
½ tsp tamari
a pinch of aonori seaweed
pomegranate seeds, optional

In one end of the box you'll already have your salad. Arrange the rice in the other end of the box (or in a whole single box, if using a double-decker like in the image) and scatter it with sesame seeds, salt and nori. In the remaining space, use a small piece of cabbage as a bowl, or separator, to arrange the sesame-fried egg and tofu. Drizzle the tamari over the tofu and scatter with aonori. Finish with pomegranate seeds, if using. Close your box and pack in a bento bag or furoshiki with a fork or chopsticks.

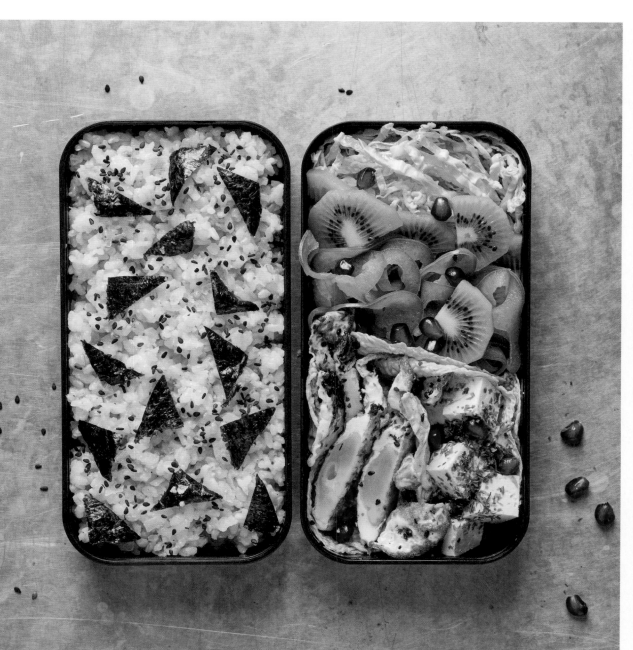

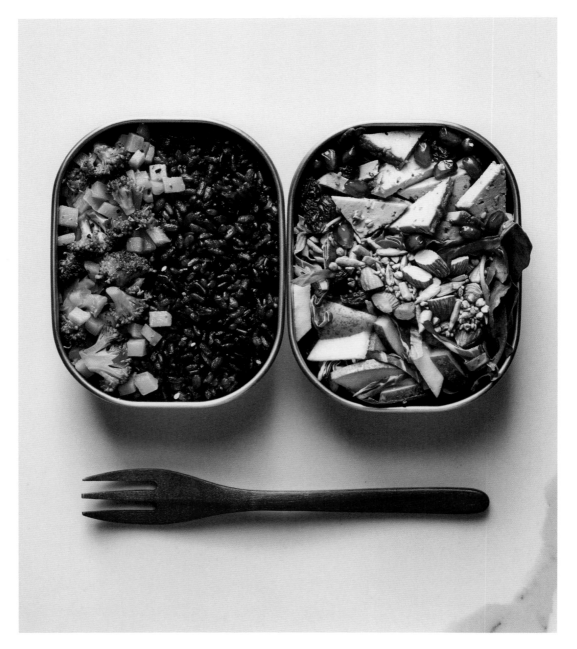

BENTO POWER

Beautiful Balance Bento

Many of my favourite combinations of flavour and texture are in this bento –
crunchy, tangy carrot-broccoli quick-pickle, naturally smoky and chewy Black
Gradient Rice (brown rice works well too), and a sweet-bitter-crunchy salad.
Like many of my bento salads, I don't use a dressing, as things tend to get a
bit messy, either at lunchtime, or when transporting the box home. Instead I
use a combination of juicy, acidic and oil-rich ingredients that merge the salad
together – like the pear, pomegranate and toasted nuts do here.

Makes 1 bento.
Fridge life: 24 hours.

Quick-pickle makes 2 portions.
Fridge life: up to 1 week.

Broccoli and Carrot Quick-pickle

4 small broccoli florets, cut into small bite-
  sized pieces
1 small carrot, cut into small cubes
1 tbsp brown rice vinegar
½ tsp sea salt
a good pinch of chilli flakes
a pinch of nigella or cumin seeds

Place all the pickle ingredients in a sturdy
plastic bag or a small bowl. Massage
everything together until juicy and
softened, 1 minute or more. If using a
bag, remove all the air and massage
through the bag (wash and reuse the
bag afterwards). Transfer leftovers to a
glass container with a lid and store in
the fridge.

TO ASSEMBLE

1 portion of pre-prepped black
  gradient rice (page 34)
1–2 radicchio leaves, shredded,
  and/or a handful of salad
  greens
1 small pear, cut into bite-sized
  pieces
50g firm smoked tofu, cut into
  bite-sized pieces
a handful of sultanas
2–3 tbsp savoury granola
  (page 43), or toasted,
  chopped almonds
pomegranate seeds or
  blueberries, to taste, optional

Arrange the rice in one end
of your box (or in one whole
single box, if using a double-
decker) and neatly arrange half
of the pickle on top. Pour some
of the pickle juice over the rice
to flavour it.

Make a bed of radicchio and/
or salad greens in the remaining
box/space. Add the pear, tofu,
sultanas and granola/nuts in
separate mounds (or all mixed
up, if you prefer). Finish with
the pomegranate or berries, if
using. Close your box and pack
in a bento bag or furoshiki with
a fork or chopsticks.

Summer Fruits Bento

This is one to make when there's an abundance of summer produce (and you just got back from your food-shopping trip!). Let your gorgeous fruit and veg chill out on a bed of seasoned rice, draped with a nori sheet and enjoy their combination of sweet, fresh and savoury. This bento is very loosely based on chirashi sushi – sushi rice with a variety of toppings arranged beautifully in a bowl or box.

Makes 1 bento.
Fridge life: 24 hours.

TIPS:
I cut my little gem lettuce like this: bunch a few leaves together and cut the bottom, thick half in thin shreds across, this makes a good 'filler'/bed, and they're easier (and more delicious) to eat, too. Leave most of the pretty top part of the leaf intact and use as separators between dishes, or to frame your bento like in the image.

Halving your tomatoes across their waist (if you imagine the stalk being their head) makes for bento-genic tomatoes when faced up.

1 portion of pre-prepped grainy Japanese, or brown short-grain rice (pages 34 and 30)
1–2 tbsp tao beach furikake or red gomashio (pages 39 and 41)
½–1 nori sheet
a few little gem lettuce leaves (see Tip)
5cm cucumber, sliced
¼ red pepper, sliced
¼ avocado, flesh scooped out or sliced
2 ripe cherry tomatoes, halved (see Tip)
1 small sliver of watermelon, peeled, de-seeded and cut into bite-sized pieces
a few cherries or a plum, pitted
a couple of blackberries (or any summer berry)
1 overnight egg (page 51), peeled and pixelated, or 50g soft-medium tofu, cubed, or a couple of spoonfuls of cooked cannellini beans
a drizzle of lazy ra-yu chilli oil (page 48), or toasted sesame oil
sea salt and chilli flakes, to taste
1–2 tbsp of any of the seasoned nuts and seeds (page 43)

Place the rice with furikake or gomashio in your bento box and combine, taste test to see how much of the seasoning you'd like to mix in. Even the rice out to a bed and cover it with one single layer of nori – depending on box size you may need ½ or 1 sheet. Fold, rip or cut it with scissors to fit.

On top of the nori, tightly arrange the veggies, fruit and egg, tofu or beans, if using, in separate sections. Drizzle a little chilli or sesame oil over the egg/tofu/beans and and add a pinch of salt too. Finish with seasoned nuts and seeds, or more furikake or gomashio if you prefer, either in a small mound, or dotted around the veggies and fruit. Close your box and pack in a bento bag or furoshiki with a fork or chopsticks.

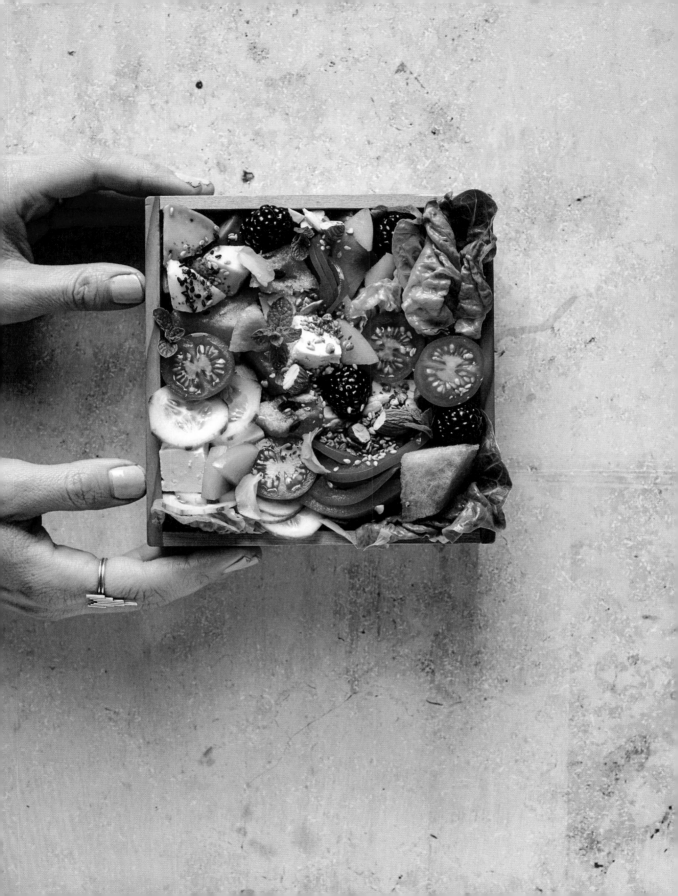

Red Velvet Quinoa Bento

This stunning quinoa is one of my most asked-for recipes on Instagram and this is the first time I share it, I hope you will like it! Beetroot, miso and a touch of clove add a sensuous, earthy quality to this quinoa, in happy company of creamy avocado, pecans and fragrant charred peach and asparagus. Stone fruit is mostly sold under-ripe to protect it from bruising – a blast of heat brings its sweetness and softness out instantly. Char it with the asparagus in a dry pan, or over a naked gas flame – a simple technique normally used to grill small green shishito peppers in Japan.

Makes 1 bento.

Red velvet quinoa makes 2–3 portions.
Fridge life: up to 3 days.
Charred peach and asparagus
makes 1 portion. Eat the same day.

Red Velvet Quinoa

200g quinoa, washed and drained
1 medium beetroot, scrubbed and roughly
   chopped into small pieces
400ml water, to cook
2 tbsp brown rice miso paste
3 tbsp extra virgin olive oil
½ tsp ground cinnamon
pinch of ground cloves (or crumble the top
   of 1 clove bud)
a little finely grated zest and juice of
   1 unwaxed lemon

Place the washed, wet quinoa in a pan and toast over a high heat, stirring frequently until it looks dry and crackles a lot (it's fine if it gets a little 'burnt', as this adds a good smoky flavour). Add the beetroot and measured water for cooking, cover and bring to the boil, then simmer over a low heat until the grains are soft and all the water is gone, 15–20 minutes. Whisk the rest of the quinoa ingredients together in a large mixing bowl, add the hot quinoa and combine well. Leave to cool slightly before packing in your bento and/or storage container with a lid. Store in the fridge.

Charred Peach and Asparagus

½ slightly under-ripe peach or nectarine
3–4 asparagus stalks, woody ends
   removed

Either use a very hot, dry frying pan and press the fruit (cut side-down) and asparagus with a spatula for a few moments to char, add a splash of water then quickly cover with a lid for a minute or two to soften them. Or, place a metal grid (I use an old oven rack) over your biggest gas flame and when it's red hot, press the peach/nectarine and then the asparagus onto the hot rack for a few seconds to get grill marks, then reduce the heat to its lowest and leave them to char for 30 seconds on each side. Transfer to a plate and leave to cool.

TO ASSEMBLE
Per Bento

a few little gem lettuce leaves
½ avocado, flesh scooped out
   or sliced
2–3 tbsp toasted pecans or
   cashew nut clusters (page 43)
½ tbsp tamari, optional
a squeeze of lime juice, optional

Arrange the quinoa in one end of your box (or in a whole box, if using a double-decker like in the image). Make a bed of lettuce in the remaining space and arrange the avocado, peach/nectarine and asparagus on top. Add the nuts, either in a divider or a pocket made from baking paper (page 116). If you want dressing, pour the tamari and a squeeze of lime juice into a small leak-proof pot to take with you and drizzle over the veggies later. Close your box and pack in a bento bag or furoshiki with the dressing pot, and a fork or chopsticks.

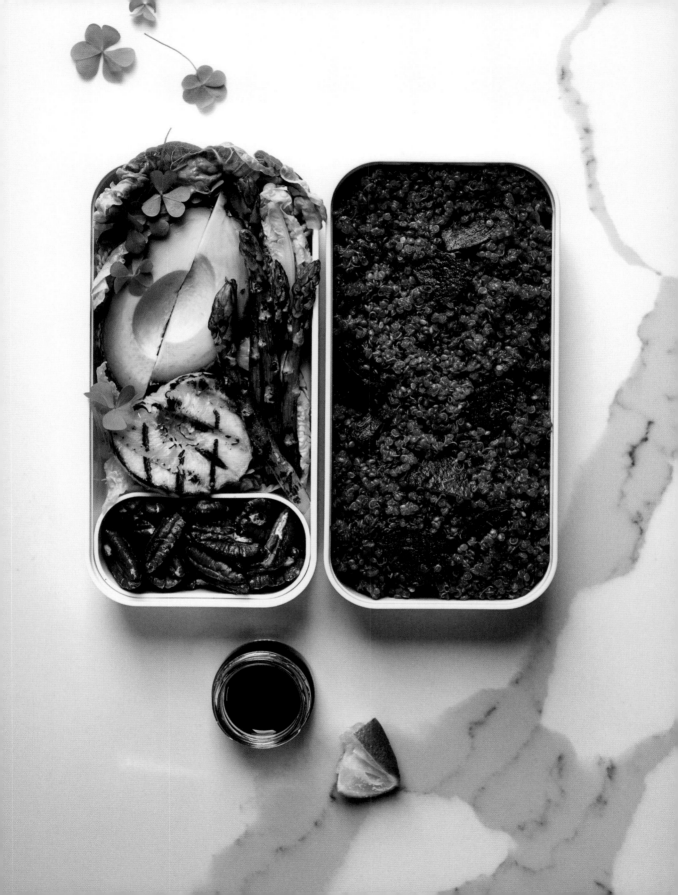

Mixed Blessings Onigiri Bento

A complete meal in one ball of blessings! I'm taking full advantage of mixed grains here; the part white rice makes the onigiri easy to shape, the part brown rice and quinoa adds nutrients and filling power and it's all finished off with nutritious watercress, seeds and pretty peas! Sanshō is a Japanese spice with a unique, slightly tongue-tingling aroma, similar to Sichuan pepper (which it can be subbed with) that really perks up rice. Depending on their freshness, the peppercorns can be very potent, so try with a small amount first. If you can't find either of these spices, just use freshly ground black pepper.

Onigiri makes 5 x 100g balls
(enough for 2–3 bento).
Fridge life: Eat the same day.

100g white Japanese rice
100g brown short-grain rice
50g quinoa
350ml water, to cook
1 bunch (about 150g) of watercress
   (stalks included), thoroughly washed
½ tsp flaky sea salt
10–15 grains of sanshō or sichuan
   pepper, crushed
200g frozen peas straight from
   the freezer
a few spoonfuls of zen pebble furikake,
   toasted sesame seeds or green
   gomashio (pages 39 and 41), optional
a small bowl of water and a small plate
   of sea salt to shape the onigiri

TO ASSEMBLE
Per Bento

1 portion of any seasoned nuts
   and seeds (pages 43–44),
   plus dried fruit or raisins
1 small carrot, peeled if needed,
   and halved lengthways

To make the onigiri, wash the combined rice and quinoa directly in your cooking pot with cold water, trying to rub off as much of the cloudy starch as you can with your fingers. Discard the water and repeat twice. Drain completely, and add the measured water for cooking. Cover and bring to the boil, then simmer over a low heat for 15 minutes. Remove from the heat and, without removing the lid, leave to stand for 5 minutes before using.

While the rice cooks, quick-blanch the watercress. Place it, stalks and all, in a heatproof bowl and pour boiling water over to submerge. Leave for 2 minutes, then drain in a strainer and cool completely under a cold running tap. Tightly squeeze it in your hands to remove as much water as possible. Chop finely and, while it's still on the chopping board, mix it with the salt and sanshō or sichuan pepper.

Dump the cooked rice/quinoa mix in a large mixing bowl and gently mix in the frozen peas – they will help cool down the mixture. It's ready to use when it's cool enough to handle with your bare hands. Gently fold in the watercress, plus optional seasonings to taste.

Part the rice into 5 equal parts. Wet, then dab your hands with a little salt (the salt both flavours and helps keep the rice fresh so don't skip this step) and gently but firmly squeeze each part of the rice into balls, wetting your hands in between each one. See overleaf for more detailed instructions. Pack a couple or so of the rice balls snugly in your bento box, or wrap each one in baking paper or reusable wrap. Pack the carrot in any remaining space in the box, or in a separate pot, and nuts and dried fruit in a small separate pot. Pack in a bento bag or furoshiki with a napkin.

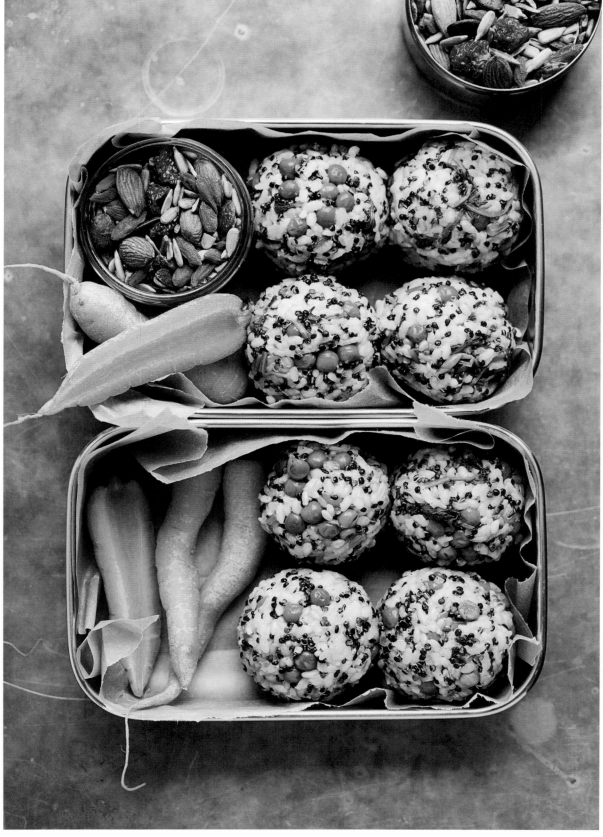

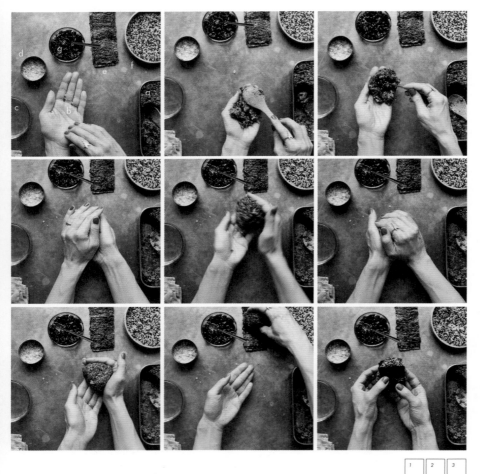

To shape Onigiri:

Get your onigiri work station ready (1):

a. Freshly cooked rice (not refrigerated), cool enough to handle with your bare hands – I often cook it the evening before and then use it the next morning
b. Thoroughly washed hands
c. A small bowl of water, to wet your hands
d. Salt, to rub your hands with
e. If you're wrapping in nori, ready-cut nori strips (see below)
f. If you are rolling in sesame or furikake, a small plate filled
g. Filling, if using

Wet your hands and rub a pinch of salt between your palms (1).

Scoop up a handful of rice. It can be any amount, just ensure it will fit both in your hand and your bento box! (2).

If you are filling your onigiri, mould a hole in your rice, then fill it (3) and hug the rice to close the hole (4).

Shape by hugging the rice rhythmically with both hands, turning after each hug so it shapes evenly (5–6). It should be firm enough to hold its shape while you eat it, but not squashed to a hard lump. To make a triangle shape, make both your hands into an L-shape, turning after each hug (7).

Wrap in a strip of nori or roll in sesame seeds or furikake (8–9).

To rip:

Fold and rip your nori just like paper. Fold (i) and carefully rip (ii). Layer the nori strips on top of each other, fold and rip again (iii). The strips can be anything from a few cm wide to as wide as your onigiri.

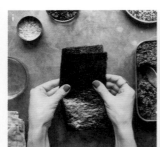
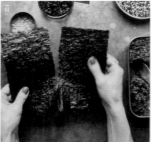
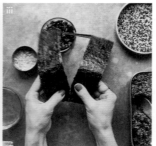

How to – Onigiri – Rice Balls

Onigiri, or oni-gary-barry as Andy calls them, is one of our bento favourites. They're hand-shaped, hand-held rice balls wrapped in nori or sesame, sometimes filled, sometimes with seasonings mixed in with the rice. The sandwich of Japan!

Onigiri is not sushi, but both were developed pre-fridge times, so their seasonings doubled up as a preservative – onigiri are shaped with damp hands rubbed with salt, which keeps them fresh for longer, whilst sushi rice is infused in a salt and vinegar seasoning liquid (which also preserves it). Wrapping onigiri in nori also helps to keep nasties out (a kind of edible food-wrap!).

For successful onigiri, use freshly cooked rice, washed and cooked right (page 29) and a gentle but firm hand when shaping. An onigiri should not be sticky (or solid) to bite into, but not fall apart either. Become friends with your rice – each grain is an individual. Ease it into a harmony with its neighbours. You can shape your onigiri into a triangle shape or ball, small or big – whatever fits into you hand, and your bento box! White Japanese rice (page 28) is the easiest to begin with and mixed-grain rice works well too (pages 34–35). Pure brown rice is more challenging to shape. Try the 50/50 rice (page 35) if you like a browner onigiri. Jasmine, basmati and other types of rice simply won't hold together.

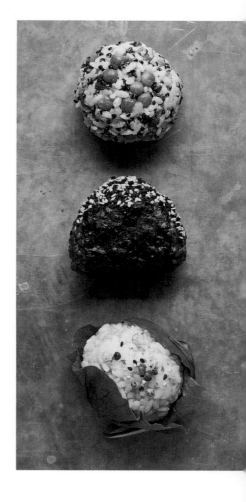

To wrap:
Onigiri are handheld so need a 'wrap' of sorts – nori is perfect for this, or roll your onigiri in sesame or furikake. Or use a shiso leaf, radicchio leaf, or any other large, thin (or lightly steamed) leaf.

To fill:
Fillings are optional and are meant to be small and concentrated, so you take a bite of rice with a small bite of filling. You can use anything you like as long as it's not very wet or oily. Some suggestions:

½ tsp miso paste (you can add some sesame seeds, or a little grated ginger to the miso paste as well)
1–2 tsp savoury granola (page 43)
½ tsp ume boshi plum paste

To store:
Eat on the same day. Keep away from wet foods in your bento box. The less they come in contact with air the better. Most Japanese recipes call for clingfilm, but I prefer plastic-free options like wax wrap, baking paper and tinfoil or simply ensuring that my onigiri fits really snugly in my box, with minimal air exposure.

Lady Power Moon Bento

I've explored ways of getting more iron and minerals into my diet my whole adult life, as I'm inherently aenemic. This bento is not just packed full of blood-boosting ingredients, but it has sweetness, pretty colours and a little chocolate treat to cheer anyone up, at any time of the month!

Makes 1 bento.
Fridge life: up to 24 hours.

Gochujang-glazed beans makes 2–3 portions.
Fridge life: up to 3 days.
Carrot ribbon quick-pickle makes 2–4 portions.
Fridge life: 1 week.

TIP:

To make a small paper-pouch to pack nuts or treats in, use a 10–15cm square of baking paper (1), fold it in half (2), fold again into a quarter (3), open up (4) and fill it up!

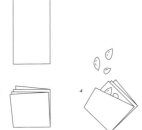

Gochujang-glazed Beans

240g red kidney beans (drained and rinsed, if using canned)
1 tbsp gochujang sauce (page 48)
2 tsp garlic-infused soy sauce (page 47)
1 tsp maple syrup
1 tsp water if needed to make a paste

Whisk together the gochujang, soy sauce, maple and water directly in an airtight storage container. Add the beans and mix to ensure they are coated well. Store leftovers in the fridge.

Carrot Ribbon Quick-pickle

1 medium carrot (100g), peeled (I use a mix of regular and purple carrot to get the red colour in the image)
1 tbsp apple cider vinegar
¼ tsp sea salt
½ tsp pink peppercorns, lightly crushed

Ribbon the carrot with a potato peeler, rotating the carrot after each long stroke (finely slice the core of the carrot and add it to the mix too), then add it along with the vinegar, salt and peppercorns directly to a glass jar with a lid and shake to combine. Store leftovers in the fridge. The flavour develops over time.

TO ASSEMBLE

1 portion of pre-prepped sister power rice (between ⅓–½ of one batch), page 37
a handful of salad greens
a handful of flat-leaved parsley
mixed nuts, seeds and dried fruit to taste
a few pieces of dark chocolate
a few raspberries, optional

Shape the rice into a few small onigiri (page 114), or leave it as it is, arranged in one end of your bento box. If you've made onigiri, I like lining my bento box with a little baking paper before packing the onigiri.

In the remaining space of your box (or your second box, if using a double-decker, like in this image), make a bed of salad greens and rest a portion of beans and quick-pickles on top. I like adding the parsley bunched up whole, to pick at, but you can also tear it and mix with the salad greens.

Add the nuts mix and chocolate in a paper pouch (see Tip) and finish with a couple of raspberries, if using. Pack everything in a bento bag or furoshiki with a fork or chopsticks.

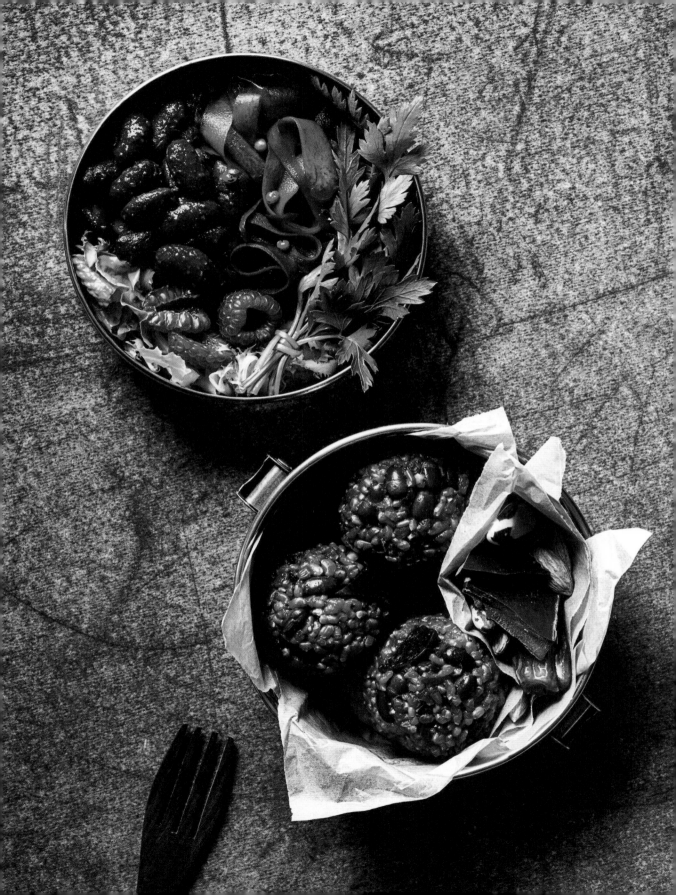

Rawmari Mushroom Bento

Massaging raw mushrooms in a tamari marinade transforms them into a fragrant, super savoury wonder in just a few moments, a little like 'mushroom sashimi' (raw fish), with juice that makes the best dressing for grains and salad veggies. It's something I often make as a 'weight' in a raw dish – dotted out over a giant salad, for example. It can be varied indefinitely, just add any herb, spice or oil along with a salty element to the marinade. Here I've combined it with quinoa for protein, a juicy, simple tomato salad (with sun-dried tomatoes that will rehydrate till lunch) and creamy pine nuts.

Makes 1 bento.
Fridge life: up to 24 hours.

Rawmari mushrooms makes
3 portions.
Fridge life: up to 4 days.

Rawmari Mushrooms

250g chestnut or button mushrooms
2 tbsp tamari
1 tbsp balsamic vinegar
½ tsp sea salt (smoked, if possible)
½ tsp Herbes de Provence or
   dried rosemary
a pinch of garlic granules, optional
½ tsp torn fresh thyme, optional

Wash the mushrooms, then cut them in roughly 5mm-thick slices. Add them to a mixing bowl with the rest of the rawmari ingredients then, using clean hands, repeatedly push down hard on the mushrooms until they are quite crushed and release a lot of liquid, about 1 minute. Set aside for assembly. (Store leftovers in a glass jar with a lid in the fridge.)

TO ASSEMBLE

1 portion pre-prepped quinoa
   (page 31)
1 big ripe tomato
1 sun-dried tomato (oil-free, or
   drained and patted dry)
½–1 tbsp extra virgin olive oil
1 tbsp pine nuts, raw or toasted
a few chives or 1 spring onion,
   finely chopped
a handful of salad greens

Use a leak-proof box or jar with a lid. Start with a layer of quinoa, topping it with a third of the mushrooms, reserving their liquid to top the tomatoes with.

Roughly chop the fresh tomato and finely shred the sun-dried tomato over it on the chopping board, using scissors (or you can use a knife). Combine the two types of tomato with your hands, then add the mixture to the bento box. Top the tomatoes with olive oil and a third of the mushroom juice.

Finish with the pine nuts and chives or spring onions, and the salad greens. Close your box and pack in a bento bag or furoshiki with a fork or spoon.

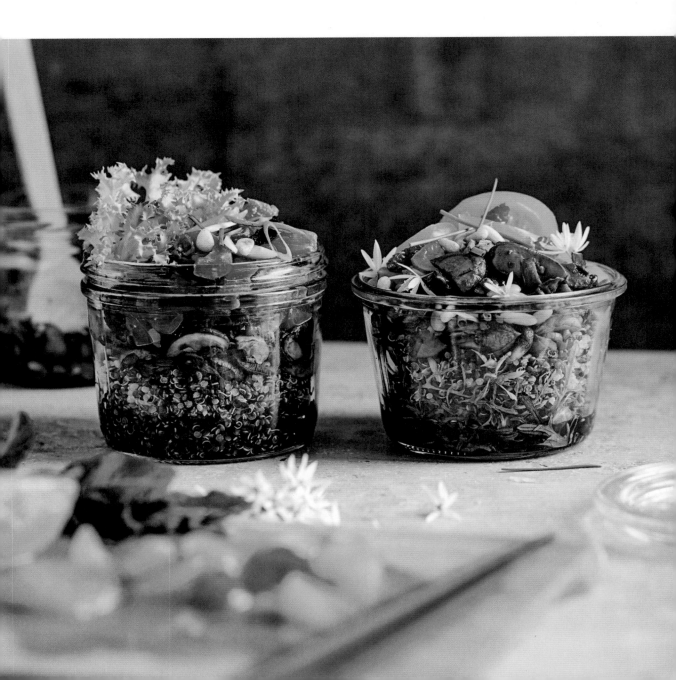

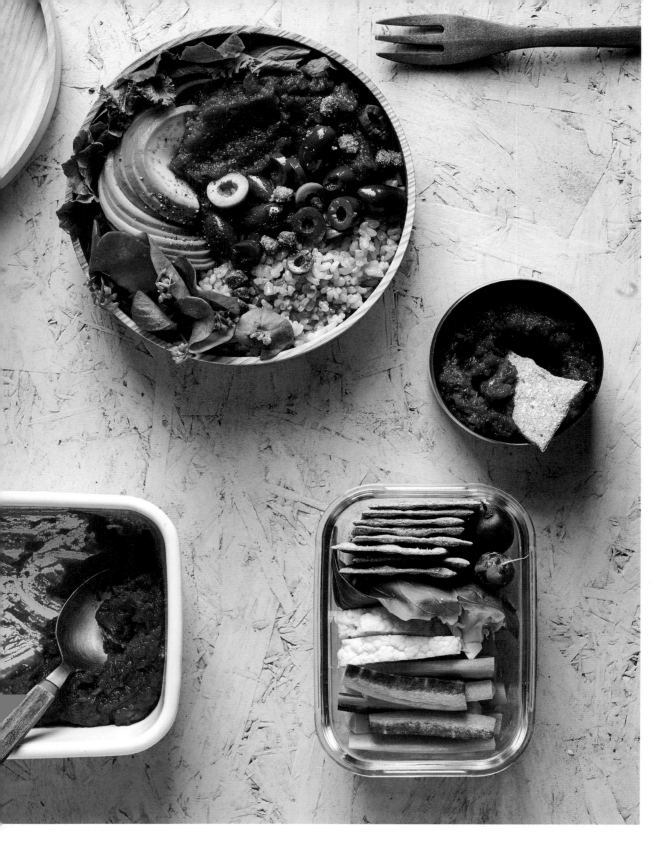

Magenta Mash Bento

This magenta-red mash is not just pretty, it's super versatile and packed with protein, fibre and mineral power from both the lentils and beetroot. I use it as something in between dhal and hummus in a bento – its subtly sweet, earthy flavour is delicious with salty, bitter and acidic flavours (olives, capers, rocket, gherkins, sauerkraut), and with brown rice. It's great as a dip with raw veggies and crackers too, or spread on toast – or even rolled into a nori roll with brown rice, a lick of miso paste and fresh coriander!

Makes 1 bento.
Fridge life: up to
2 days.

Magenta mash
makes 2–3 portions.
Fridge life: up to
4 days.

Magenta Mash

100g dried split red lentils
1 small to medium beetroot (about 100g), scrubbed
1 small red onion, roughly chopped
½ tsp sea salt
1 bay leaf or 1 clove
350ml water, to cook
2 tsp balsamic vinegar

Wash the lentils in cold water and drain completely. Place them in a pan and coarsely grate the beetroot straight into the pan, using a box- or microplane grater. Add the onion, salt, bay leaf or clove, and the measured water. Cover and bring to the boil, then simmer over a low heat for 20 minutes, until the water is absorbed and the lentils look big and mushy.

Remove the bay leaf/clove, add the vinegar and vigorously stir to create a mash. If it looks too wet, boil it over a medium heat for 1–2 minutes, stirring all the time. When you can see the bottom of the pan while stirring it's done – and as it cools it will firm up. Remove from the heat and leave to cool before using in recipes or packing as a side dish. Store in an airtight container in the fridge.

Simplest Bento Bowl

1 portion of pre-prepped quick-cook brown short-grain rice (page 30)
1 tsp flaxseed oil
1 tsp tamari
a handful of rocket, watercress or flat-leaf parsley
1 portion (about ⅓–½ batch) of magenta mash
½ avocado, flesh scooped out or sliced
1 overnight egg (page 51), halved, optional
pitted Kalamata olives, to taste
a few salted capers
freshly ground black pepper, to taste

Make a bed of rice in your bento box or bowl and drizzle with the flaxseed oil and tamari, if using. Arrange the leaves, mash, avocado and egg, if using, on top. Finish by scattering the olives (roughly chopped or left whole) and capers over the mash and a twist of black pepper. Close your box and pack in a bento bag or furoshiki with a fork.

Winter Jewels Bento

This bento's bright colours and sweet flavours, and the power of cold-weather-resistant kale and parsnip should cheer up any grey day. You can choose to make the salad in the evening and let it marinate overnight in a mixing bowl, or you can pack it in your bento box right after you've made it. It gets more and more delicious the longer the flavours merge. With roasted hazelnuts and protein-rich quinoa you're set up for a good afternoon!

Makes 2 bento.
Fridge life: up to 2 days.

Winter jewels salad makes
2 portions.
Fridge life: up to 3 days.

Winter Jewels Salad

50g kale leaves (about 6), any type, thoroughly washed
50g red cabbage, finely shredded
½ small parsnip, peeled and cut into thin half-moons
1 small carrot, peeled and cut into thin discs
30g (about 4 small) dates, finely chopped
1 orange, scrubbed and halved
2cm piece fresh ginger
½ tsp sea salt

To make the salad, rip the kale leaves off their stems and roughly chop the leaves. Unless the stalks are very dry and fibrous, chop them too, very finely, and add both the leaves and stalks either to a mixing bowl or a sturdy plastic bag, along with the rest of the salad veggies and dates. Squeeze the juice of half the orange into the mix and finely grate a little orange zest in, too. Save the second half to use later. Finely grate the ginger and hand-squeeze it over the salad mix to extract the juice (discard the pulp). Add the salt and gently massage the mix with your hands, until quite a lot of juice is released. If using a bag, remove all the air and massage through the bag (wash and reuse the bag afterwards).

Either pack in your box straight away or store in a glass container with a lid in the fridge. The more tightly packed (less air) salads like this one are stored, the better they will marinate (and slower they will spoil), so use the smallest storage container it will fit in to.

TO ASSEMBLE
Per Bento

1 portion of pre-prepped quinoa, cooled (page 31)
1 tbsp hazelnuts, toasted
1–2 tbsp saltwater nuts and seeds (page 44), or toasted almonds
1 tsp zen pebble furikake (page 38), optional
pomegranate seeds, to taste, optional

Make a bed, or slope, of quinoa in your box. Arrange the salad on top, making sure to add all of its marinating juice, too. Use a sharp knife to peel and cut the remaining half orange into bite-sized pieces, and top the salad with it. Add the nuts (or pack the nuts in a separate small container to scatter over before eating). Finish with furikake and pomegranate, if using. Close your box and pack in a bento bag or furoshiki with a fork or chopsticks.

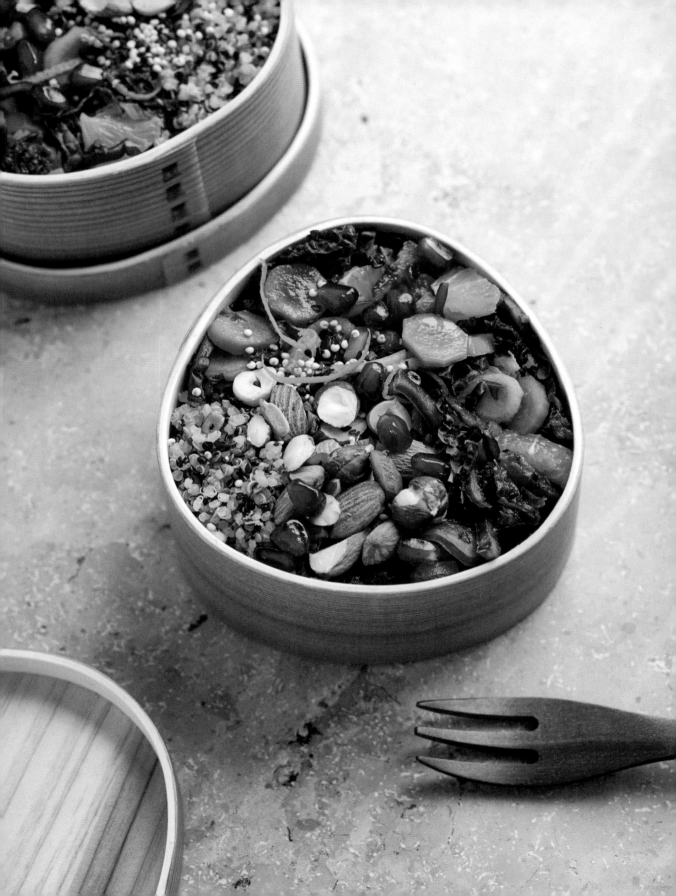

Midnight Magic Pumpkin Bento

Even if you had to run to catch your ride home from the party, there should still be time to prep this before bed – and wake up to pumpkin ready to go into your bento box! Midnight magic pumpkin is based on my memories of 'nimono' a Japanese home cooking classic. Veggies are slowly simmered in a savoury-sweet broth, where they deeply absorb flavour. I'm doing a shortcut here, letting my pumpkin finish on after-heat overnight, which allows it to slowly season without getting mushy or me watching a pot for ages! I love the result, the flavour really takes me back to Japan. You can make the recipe with any pumpkin or squash.

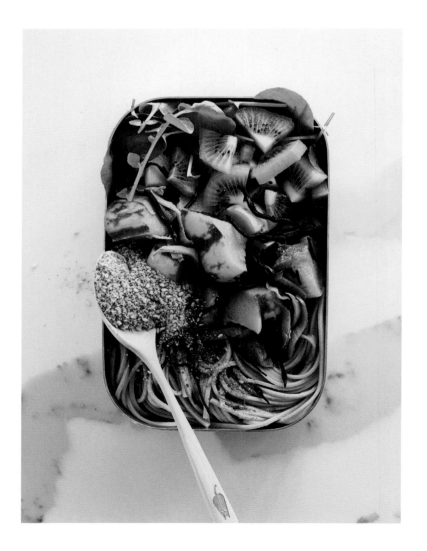

Makes 1 bento.
Fridge life: up to 24 hours.

Pumpkin makes 1–2 portions.
Fridge life: up to 4 days.

Midnight Magic Pumpkin

300g (about ½) small pumpkin or squash, peeled if thick-skinned and deseeded, cut into thick (2cm) slices
3cm piece fresh ginger, thickly sliced (5mm)
3g dried hijiki (1 big pinch) or 1 tsp instant dried wakame seaweed
1 tbsp tamari

In the evening before you assemble your bento, place the pumpkin, ginger and seaweed in a frying pan and add water to about 3cm deep, ensuring the ginger and seaweed are in the water. Drizzle the tamari over the pumpkin. Cover, bring to the boil, then simmer over a low heat for 10 minutes. If it looks like it's drying up, add more water. Turn the heat off, cover with a tea towel to keep warm and leave to finish overnight. In the morning, cut the pumpkin into bite-sized chunks and thinly shred the ginger slices.

TO ASSEMBLE

1 portion (85g) dry soba
  noodles
handful of watercress
½ kiwi, peeled and sliced, or
  flesh scooped out
gomashio or toasted sesame
  seeds, to taste (pages 40–41
chilli, to taste (shichimi togarashi
  is ideal)

Cook the soba noodles
according to the packet's
instructions. Drain in a strainer
and cool completely under
a cold running tap. Either let
the noodles drip-dry in the
strainer for 5 minutes or
instantly spin them dry in a
sturdy salad spinner.

Arrange the noodles on one
side of your bento box and
the watercress on the other. In
the middle, scoop in as much
pumpkin as you want and pour
any remaining cooking liquid
over the noodles to season.
Arrange the kiwi on top of the
watercress, add a generous pile
of gomashio or toasted sesame
on the noodles and finish with a
chilli sprinkle.

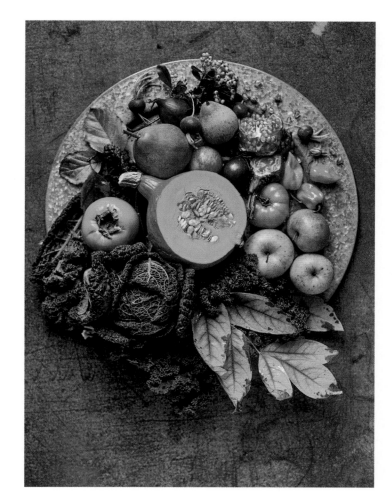

Smashed Wakame Beans Bento

Smashed wakame beans may sound unusual but they are so good, especially in a summer bento! The inspiration comes from 'su-no-mono', a Japanese side dish of vinegared cucumber and seaweed (page 152). I've made it into a protein dish by adding neutral-tasting white beans, smashed by shaking everything together in a glass jar. Once you've taken what you need out for your bento, the jar goes into the fridge, ready to use for a few days. Here they are with a favourite flavour-and-colour-combo: avocado, mango and black gradient rice.

Makes 1 bento.
Fridge life: up to 24 hours.

Smashed wakame beans makes 2–3 portions.
Fridge life: up to 4 days.

Smashed Wakame Beans

1 tbsp instant dried wakame seaweed
½ cucumber, peeled if desired
240g cooked cannellini beans (drained and rinsed, if using canned)
1 tbsp brown rice vinegar
½ tbsp coconut palm sugar
½ tbsp toasted (black) sesame seeds (page 41)
finely grated zest from ¼ unwaxed lemon (see Tip)
½ tsp sea salt
pinch of gochugaru (Korean red pepper), or chilli flakes, optional

Add the wakame to a bowl with plenty of cold water and leave it to semi-rehydrate for 3–4 minutes (so that it can still soak up some of the liquid that will release from the cucumber later), then drain and squeeze with your hands to remove as much liquid as possible.

Halve the cucumber lengthways and remove the seeds with a small spoon. Halve each half again lengthways, and then again (you'll end up with 8 long pieces). Cut into small (2–3cm) chunks.

Add the cucumber, wakame, beans and the rest of the smashed bean ingredients to a big glass jar with a lid, close tight and give it a really good shake. (Store leftovers in the fridge.)

TO ASSEMBLE

1 portion of pre-prepped black gradient rice or grainy Japanese rice (see page 34)
a handful of salad leaves
¼ avocado, flesh scooped out or sliced
a slice of mango, peeled, and thinly sliced, to taste
green gomashio (page 41) or wakame-san furikake (page 39), to taste
a few goji berries, for colour, optional

Arrange the rice in one end of your box (or in one single box, if using a double-decker box like in the image) and beans in the other end. Line the middle space with salad leaves and arrange the avocado and mango on top. Finish with gomashio or furikake in a pile on the rice, and goji berries, if using. Close your box and pack in a bento bag or furoshiki with a fork or chopsticks.

TIP:

If you're lucky enough to find yuzu powder or juice (a unique-tasting Japanese citrus), use ½ tsp dried yuzu powder or juice instead of lemon zest.

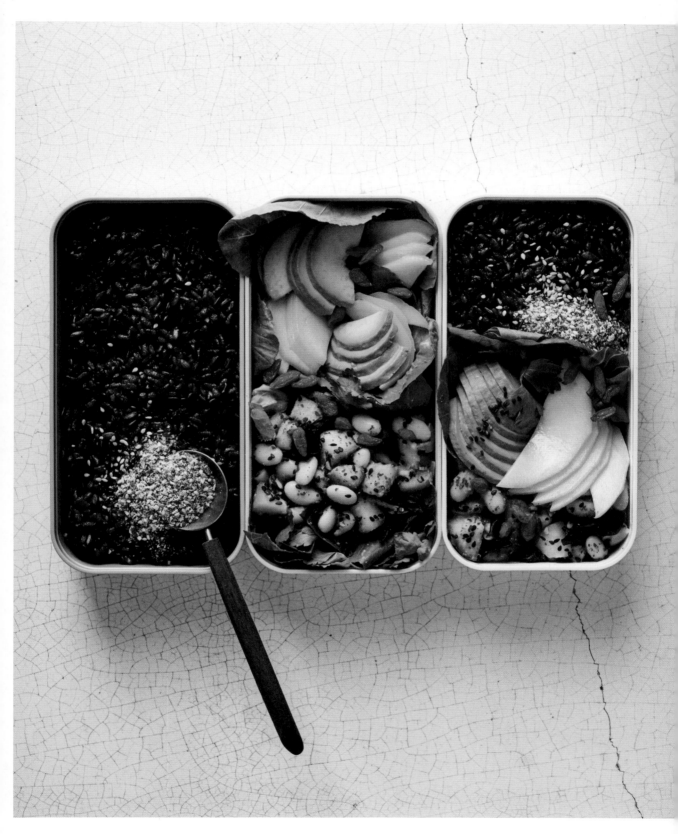

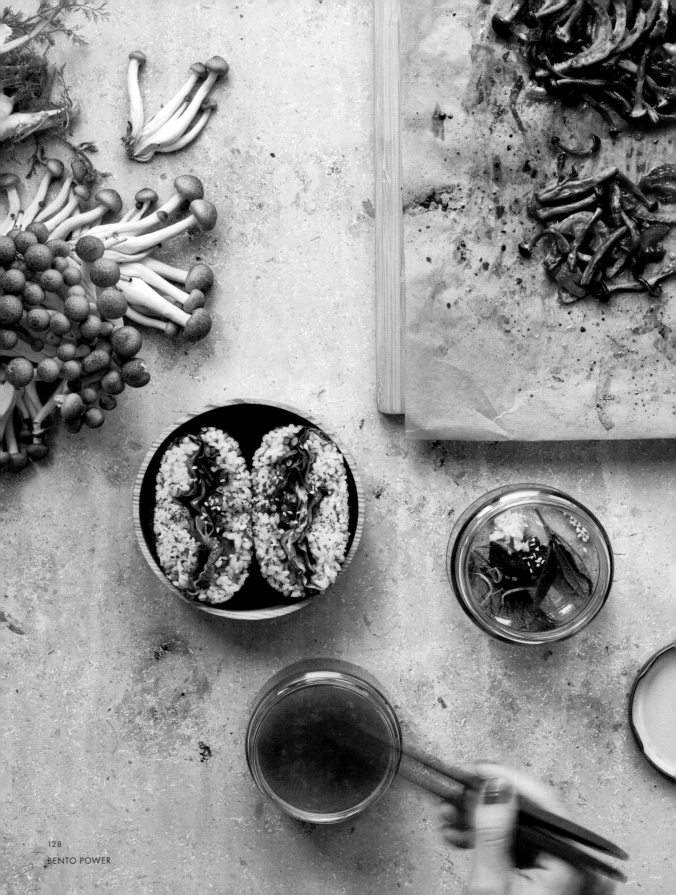

Umami-bomb Onigirazu and DIY Instant Miso Soup

Out of all the onigirazu (sushi sandwich) fillings I've made, this is my current favourite. Shimeji mushrooms are used a lot in Japan, they're tender and nutty when cooked and their stems have a really unique bite to them. I've combined them with fennel here and roasted them in the oven to concentrate their umami even more. I buy shimeji in my local greengrocer or Asian supermarkets, but if you can't find them, use button mushrooms instead, sliced.

Makes 2 bento (makes 2 big onigirazu).
Eat the same day.

Umami-bomb mix makes 2 portions.
Fridge life: up to 4 days.

DIY instant miso soup makes 1 portion
Fridge life: up to 5 days (if not using fresh herbs).

Umami-bomb Mix

1 cluster (about 150g) shimeji mushrooms, muddy ends trimmed off, or 200g button mushrooms, trimmed and sliced
1 small head of fennel, or 3 celery sticks, finely sliced on the diagonal
1½ tbsp fish sauce (vegetarian) or 2 tbsp tamari
1 tbsp light oil
½ tsp gochugaru (Korean pepper) or a good pinch of chilli flakes

Preheat the oven to 180°C/350°F/ gas mark 4. Line a large baking tray with baking paper.

Separate the shimeji mushrooms that still cluster together. Halve the fennel lengthways, then slice across their grain into very thin half moons. Add the mushrooms, fennel (or celery, if using) and the rest of the umami-bomb ingredients to the lined baking tray and mix with your hands to coat evenly. Spread the mix out thinly and roast on the highest shelf in the oven for 10–15 minutes until the mix is no longer wet, the fennel is soft and everything looks a little tanned. Remove from the oven and leave it to cool slightly before using. Wrap up any leftovers with the baking paper (like a fish and chip parcel) and store in an airtight container in the fridge.

DIY Instant Miso Soup

1 tsp brown rice miso paste
a few fine grates of fresh ginger (use a normal box grater)
a pinch of dried chilli flakes

Add-ons, optional
½ tsp instant dried wakame seaweed
fresh herbs, like dill, mint or basil, to taste
1 tbsp rolled jumbo oats (adds body and creaminess)
a pinch of garlic granules
a few grates of unwaxed lemon or orange zest

Add all the ingredients (including any add-ons, if using) to a small container, or use a slightly bigger container with enough room to make the soup in (I like using a 250ml repurposed glass jar, like in the image). When you are ready to have your soup, either tip the contents into a mug (if using a small container) or add a splash of hot water from the kettle directly to your container. Whisk with a fork or chopsticks to dissolve the miso. Top up with more hot water and your soup is ready.

TO ASSEMBLE
Per Bento

1 nori sheet
150g pre-prepped grainy Japanese rice (page 34)
½ batch of umami-bomb mix
1–2 little gem lettuce leaves
a piece of fruit of choice

Make the onigirazu according to the instructions overleaf, using the umami-bomb mix and a couple of lettuce leaves as the filling.

Either pack the onigirazu as it is, as a large closed sandwich, or cut it in half and pack in a small box, with the fruit and DIY instant miso soup on the side, in a bento bag or furoshiki with a napkin.

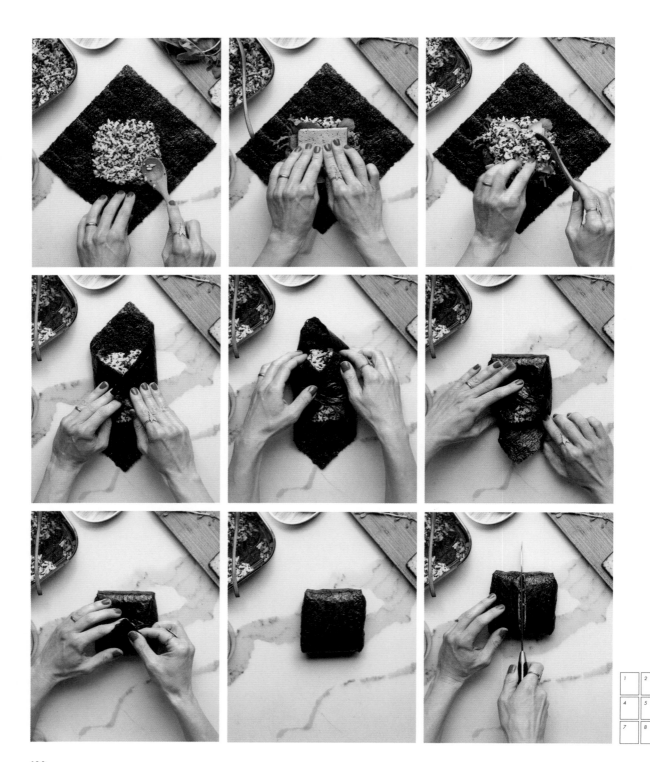

How to – Onigirazu – Sushi Sandwich

To make:
Place a nori sheet in front of you on a clean work surface, with one corner pointing towards you. Use 150g–200g rice per onigirazu. Using half of this volume (3-4 heaped tablespoons), make a square layer of rice in the middle of the nori, max 2cm thick and about 8cm square (1). Leave a little margin around the edge so you have enough nori to fold later. You can wet your hands a little to help shape the rice.

Add the fillings, as evenly as possible, and give everything a little squeeze from the top to compact (2). Finish with the second volume of rice, making a layer the same thickness as the first (3). Again, wet your hands to help shape the rice here.

To wrap:
Imagine wrapping a birthday gift. Pull the left and right nori corners together and overlap them with the filling safe inside (4). If you're using warm rice, it should be enough to glue the nori corners together, but if not, wet your hands. Do the same with the top and bottom corners (5), tucking the folded corners in to ensure that no rice peeks out (image 6–7). Flip the onigirazu over and let it rest a few minutes on your work surface for the warm rice/ water to glue the nori together (8).

To pack:
Pack the onigirazu just like it is and eat it like a sandwich, or slice in half with a sharp, wet knife to show off the pretty insides (9). You can also wrap the onigirazu, and skip on the box entirely. I use a wax wrap, or tin foil lined with baking paper, to reduce the use of plastic. Don't let damp foods touch the onigirazu if you pack it in a box, as they may dissolve the nori.

> *TIP:*
> To heat rice microwave-free use a ordinary steamer basket, lined with a little baking paper to stop the rice from falling through. Steam for 5 minutes, until piping hot.

The onigirazu or 'sushi sandwich' is a contemporary sibling to the onigiri and a brilliant invention: rice plus whatever fillings you like, folded into a whole nori sheet like a parcel. You don't need to be a pro to get it right straight away and you can get enough filling in there for a substantial lunch (I make 1–2 onigirazu per person).

Use white Japanese (page 29), brown short-grain (page 30) or any mixed-grain rice (pages 34–35) to make onigirazu. If you use the rice warm, its steam 'glues' the nori wrap together. If you use room temperature rice, use wet hands to wrap, to make it stick that way. Onigirazu is best made in the morning with fresh rice and eaten the same day, but you can make it in the evening and refrigerate it overnight too (but you'll have drier rice). Once you've got the hang of parcelling it up (doesn't take long), they can easily become a lunch staple.

Go wild with the fillings! You'll soon work out how much your onigirazu can hold before it's impossible to close. Use anything as long as it's not too wet or oily. Just ensure you always finish with a top layer of rice, so that no moist filling touches (and dissolves) the seaweed.

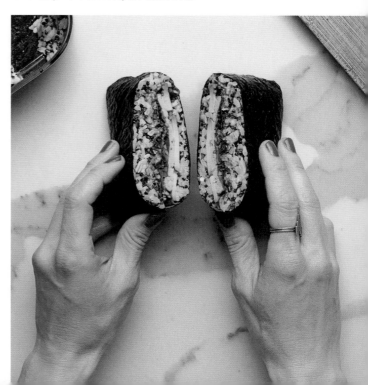

Tamago-yaki Bento and Seed Omelette Bento

'Tamago-yaki' really is one of the most classic bento fillings, so much so that some think it's not a real bento if it's not in there! You may have tried it as sushi – a neat, yellow and often very sweet omelette slice. My version is a lot less sweet and less complicated to make and I've cut out the more difficult-to-source ingredients. See overleaf for how to make it.

To make a plant-based alternative to Tamago-yaki, I experimented with millet, which has a lovely yellow colour and a decent protein count. Soaking the seed (which I do for this 'omelette') you could say, at least symbolically, it is a plant's equivalent of an egg – the beginning of their offspring, activated (by water) and ready to grow into a plant! It needs a long soak (best overnight) to work or it will break in the pan.

Makes 1 portion.
Fridge life: 3 days.

Seed Omelette

3 tbsp millet
1 tbsp golden linseeds
100ml water
2 tsps tamari
¼ tsp baking powder
½ tsp extra virgin olive oil, to fry
a couple of sprigs of flat-leaf parsley or
   dill, finely chopped, optional
black pepper, to taste

TIP:
Leftover seed omelette is surprisingly delicious shredded in a stir-fry.

Soak the millet and linseeds and measured water overnight. Without draining the water, add tamari and baking powder, and blend on high until very smooth (a small blender jug works best). Heat a frying pan over a medium-high heat, drizzle with a little oil and pour all the batter in, spreading it out like a crepe. Cook for 2–3 minutes, until brown underneath and it seems to hold together enough to flip. Flip carefully as it is more delicate than an egg omelette, and cook for a further 2–3 minutes, until brown and still a little moist inside.

If it seems like it may burn at any point, turn the heat down a little (the omelette likes it quite hot, so not too low). Transfer to a chopping board. To get the swirl effect seen in the image, scatter the parsley and pepper all over the omelette, then, starting from one end, firmly roll it into a roll. Or, use gomashio (page 41) instead of herbs. Let it cool slightly before cutting into 4cm pieces, short enough to fit into your box, standing on one end like in the image and pack immediately (or they may unravel!). Store leftovers in an airtight container in the fridge.

TO ASSEMBLE
Per Bento

1 portion of pre-prepped farm
   rice (page 36), or any rice
a handful of salad greens
2–3 slices tamago-yaki
   (recipe overleaf), or 1 seed
   omelette
a few cherry tomatoes
1 radish, thinly sliced (use a
   mandolin if you have one)
1 fig, halved
1–2 tbsp savoury granola
   (page 43)
toasted black sesame seeds
   (page 41), to taste

Fill one side of your bento box with rice. In the remaining space, make a bed of lettuce, then arrange the tamago-yaki slices, or rolled seed omelette on top. Add the cherry tomatoes, radish, fig and savoury granola in separate mounds and finish with a sprinkle of sesame seeds. Close your box and pack in a bento bag or furoshiki with a fork or chopsticks.

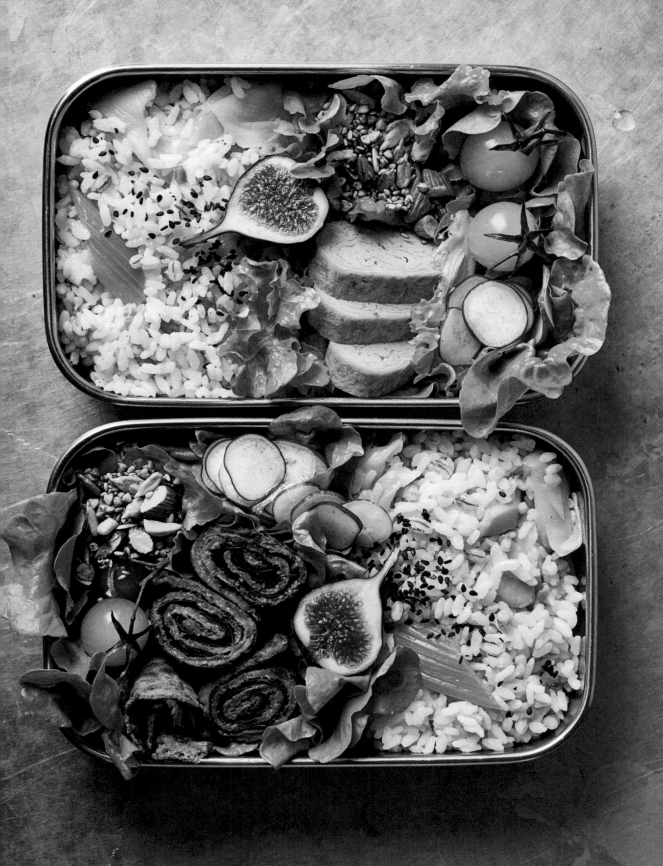

How to Tamago-yaki – Rolled Omelette, Shiso-style

Apart from being a delicious bento favourite, I see Tamago-yaki as a brilliant 'log' of protein, that lasts surprisingly long in the fridge (wrapped carefully) and you cut as you go through the week (like you would a loaf of bread). I've listed two eggs in the recipe, but mostly I make it with 3–4 eggs as it keeps so well – and the thicker the tamago-yaki, the easier it is to roll in the frying pan.

Tamago-yaki makes 2 portions.
Fridge life: up to 5 days.

Tamago-yaki Omelette

2 organic large eggs
2 tbsp water
½ tsp tamari
pinch of fine sea salt
1 tsp coconut palm sugar or ½ tsp normal sugar or agave syrup, optional
a little oil, to fry

TIP:
As you get more confident with your Tamago-yaki, try laying ½ nori sheet between some of your batter layers, just before rolling them up. Or mix frozen thawed peas into the batter.

Add all the tamago-yaki ingredients, except the oil for frying, to a glass jar with a lid, close it tight and give it a really good shake (1). Preheat a small to medium size frying pan over a medium to hight heat and then rub with a little oil (use a wad of kitchen towel like in image 5 for a thin, even coating). You are now going to make several crepe-shaped layers of omelette, each folded around the previous layer, a little like a flattened Swiss roll.

Pour a first, thin layer of batter into the pan (2) and tilt to cover the whole surface, just like a crepe. Loosen the edges with a spatula and, just as it starts looking matt, fold it over a few times (3–4). The fold shouldn't be more than about 5cm wide.

Rub the pan with oil between each layer (5). With the roll pushed to one end of the pan, pour your next layer in as before (6). It is best if you can get the batter under the roll too, so lift one side of it and tilt the pan to run the batter underneath (7). This will 'glue' the next layer to the existing roll. Once the second crepe is just about getting matt, start from your existing roll and fold it over the new layer, pressing down a little after each roll to stick (8). Rub the pan with oil again, then repeat until you have run out of batter.

Slide your roll onto a square of baking paper (9). While the tamago is still hot, it is malleable – take advantage of this and roll it up firmly in the paper (10), to get the classic tamago shape. Push the edges of the tamago in, too, to give it a good shape (11).

Traditionally, a sushi bamboo rolling mat is used for this, but I use baking paper as it lets the tamago-yaki cool while letting steam escape and still keeping moisture in – and it's practical to store it folded up just like that (12) in the fridge, too.

If you are using the tomago-yaki right away in a bento, let it cool slightly before cutting or it may break.

Leave the tomago-yaki to cool completely before storing it in the fridge. Don't pre-cut it, as it will spoil faster.

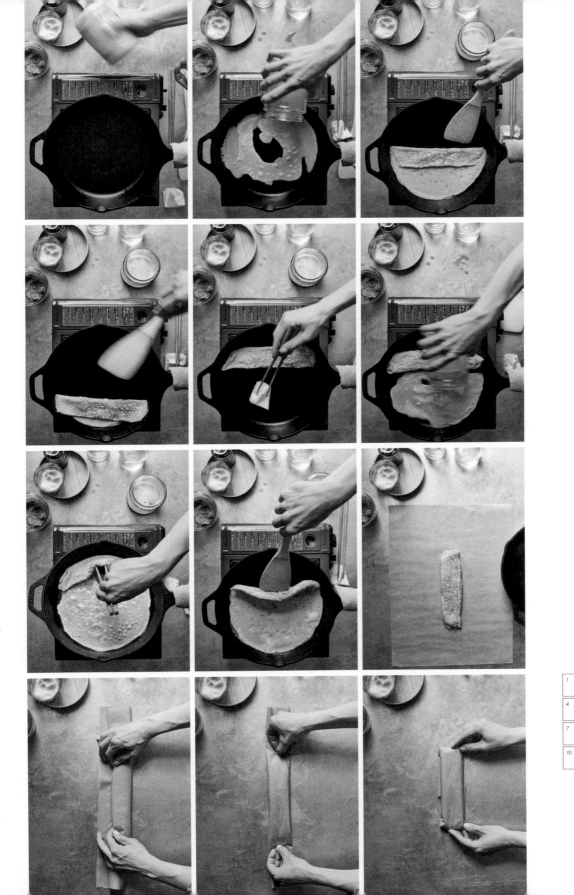

Zen Bento

Once in a while I like sprouting my rice. It's a lot less intimidating than it sounds and it's delicious! Sprouting boosts nutritional value and improves texture – and brings me back to my more 'hardcore' veggie days (when I sprouted *everything!*). Sprouting takes 1–2 days (hence the 'zen') and only works with brown rice (the beginning of the sprout is the tiny white fleck at the end of each dry grain). I've added mung beans to the rice as they are one of the easiest pulses to sprout and add interest and extra protein. The carrots, beans and tofu are just 'cut, season and go'.

Makes 1 bento.
Fridge life 24 hours.

Zen rice makes 2–3 portions.
Fridge life: up to 3 days.

Zen Rice

220g brown short-grain rice
4 tbsp dried mung beans
350ml water, to cook
1 tbsp brown rice vinegar
2 tbsp black gomashio (page 41)
½ tsp sea salt

Place the rice and beans in a bowl, cover with plenty of cold water and leave to soak overnight. The next day, drain the rice and beans, then leave them sitting in a colander over a big bowl on your worktop, covered with a clean, double-folded tea towel. Don't let them dry out, and rinse thoroughly under a cool tap twice every 24 hours (you can use filtered water if you prefer).

Depending on your room temperture, tiny tails will start emerging on the grains and beans after ½–1 day, or a little more. Either cook them now (see below) or wait another day or so to grow them longer (just keep them clean and moist by rinsing). They should smell fresh and not alcoholic or unpleasant.

To cook, rinse the rice mix in fresh water, drain, then add to your cooking pot, along with the measured water for cooking. Cover with a lid and bring to the boil, then simmer over a low heat for 20 minutes (or white rice setting if using a rice cooker).

Remove from the heat and, without removing the lid, leave to stand for 10 minutes. While still warm, fold in the vinegar, gomashio and salt, taking care not to crush the grains or tails too much. Let it cool slightly before packing in your bento box.

Carrot Chopping Board Quick-pickle

1 small-medium carrot, washed and peeled
1 tbsp goji berries or raisins
1 tsp brown rice vinegar
a pinch of sea salt

Cut the carrot into bite-sized chunks and, while it's still on your chopping board, add the goji berries or raisins, vinegar and salt and mix briefly with your hands to combine with the carrot.

TO ASSEMBLE

a handful of salad leaves
3–4 runner/flat beans, cut into bite-sized pieces on the diagonal, immersed in boiling water for 5 minutes then rinsed cold
50g soft-medium tofu, cubed
½ ripe tomato, roughly chopped
fresh bird's eye chilli, finely chopped, to taste
1 tsp tamari
a drizzle of lazy ra-yu chilli oil (page 48), or toasted sesame oil
toasted sesame seeeds (page 41), to taste

Arrange one portion of the zen rice in one end of your box and make a bed of salad leaves in the remaining space. Arrange the beans and the carrot quick-pickle in separate mounds on top. The carrots will marinate ('pickle') slightly until lunchtime. Use a salad leaf as a bowl for the tofu and top it with chopped tomatoes, chilli, tamari and oil. Finish with a sprinkle of sesame seeds. Close your box and pack in a bento bag or furoshiki with a fork or chopsticks.

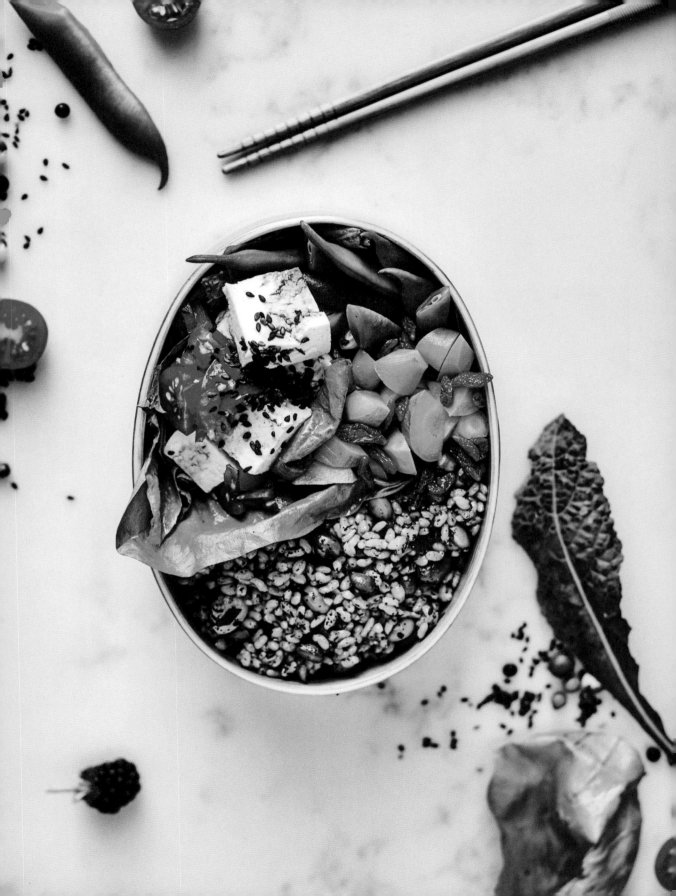

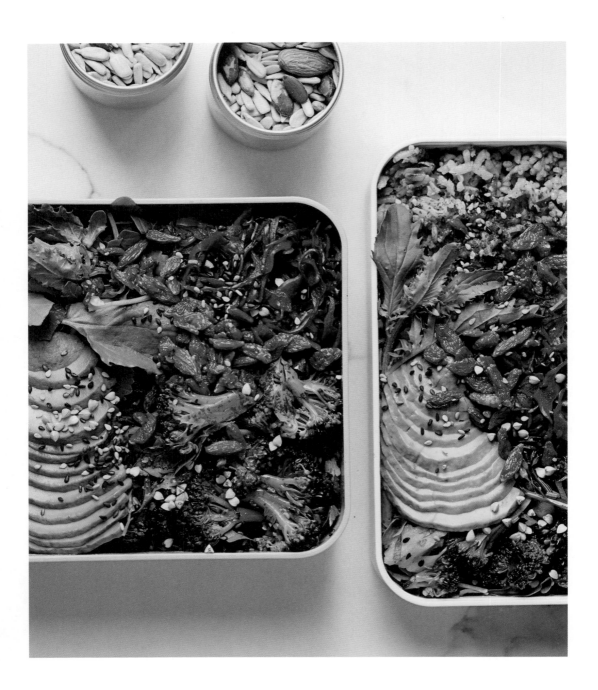

Purple and Green Quick-pickle Bento

I've made versions of this cabbage and broccoli for years – they're both true Sara classics! The broccoli can be quick-pickled raw, but I like how quick-blanching if first takes its rough edge off and lets it absorb the marinade better. These tangy, crunchy and slightly bitter pickles are balanced by creamy avocado and sweet dried fruit. I like to rinse my dried fruit briefly under the tap (just simply, in my hand), not just to clean them (as I would any fruit or veggie) but to moisten too, so by lunchtime they've rehydrated just a little (= woken up!).

Makes 1 bento.

Purple quick-pickle and
Green quick-pickle both make
around 4 portions.
Fridge life: 1 week or more.

Purple Quick-pickle (Gingery Cabbage)

¼ medium (200g) red cabbage (see Tip), very finely shredded
4cm piece fresh ginger, washed but not peeled, finely grated
1 tbsp umesu seasoning or 1 tsp sea salt
1 tbsp brown rice vinegar
a couple of scrapes of unwaxed lemon zest

Place the cabbage in a sturdy plastic bag or a small bowl. Hand-squeeze the ginger over (discard the pulp), then add the remaining ingredients. Massage everything together until juicy and softened, a minute or more. If using a bag, remove all the air and massage through the bag (wash and reuse the bag afterwards). Transfer the leftovers to a glass container with a lid and store in the fridge.

Green Quick-pickle (Broccoli)

100g broccoli (regular or sprouting), florets separated, halved and cut into bite-sized chunks
finely grated zest and juice of ½ unwaxed lemon
1 tbsp tamari
½ tsp coconut palm sugar
¼ tsp pink peppercorns

To quick-blanch your broccoli, place it in a heatproof bowl and pour boiling water over to submerge. Leave for 5 minutes, drain, then add it hot to a storage container with a lid, along with the rest of the broccoli-pickling ingredients. Toss to mix. It's best left overnight, or at least until it has cooled down, to absorb the seasonings. Store in the fridge.

TO ASSEMBLE

1 portion pre-prepped black gradient rice (page 34), see Tip
a handful of rocket or watercress
½ avocado, flesh scooped out or sliced
a generous handful of sultanas or goji berries, briefly washed under a tap
a generous handful of saltwater-toasted nuts and seeds (page 44), or any toasted nuts and seeds

Make a bed of rice in your bento box. Arrange a portion each of the cabbage, broccoli, green leaves, avocado and dried fruit in separate sections on top of the rice and make sure to pour some of the marinating juices in, too. Pack the nuts and seeds either in a small container to the side (to sprinkle over before eating) or directly on top of the ingredients. Close your box and pack in a bento bag or furoshiki with a fork or chopsticks.

TIPS:
You can use white cabbage or green cabbage like hispi, in place of red.

To get the lilac rice tint in the image, cook black gradient rice according to instructions on page 34, but use 240g white rice and just 20g black rice.

Chick'n Peas and Dandelion Greens Bento

––––––

Have you ever picked dandelion greens for your salad? It's like having your own home-grown produce, but skipping on the gardening! Dandelion leaves have a slightly bitter flavour (a little similar to rocket), delicious mixed with salad greens and best picked as new leaves in early spring. If you pick them later in the year, choose the newest, most tender part of the plant. Avoid picking near busy roads and wash the leaves thoroughly before using. Chick'n Peas really taste a bit like chicken (depending on the kind of chickpeas you use). They're pretty irresistible straight out of the oven, but they keep so well it's worth doubling the batch.

Makes 1 bento.
Fridge life: up to 2 days.

Chick'n peas makes
1–3 portions.
Fridge life: up to 4 days.

Chick'n Peas

240g cooked chickpeas (drained and
  rinsed, if using canned), briefly dried
  in a clean tea towel
1 tbsp olive oil
¼ tsp whole cumin seeds
¼ tsp garlic granules
1 squeeze of fresh lemon juice
½ tsp sea salt (smoked flaky sea salt,
  if possible)
20g flat-leaf parsley, finely chopped
½ tsp chilli flakes or gochugaru
  (Korean pepper)

Preheat the oven to 180°C/350°F/gas mark 4 and line a big baking tray with baking paper.

Pile the chickpeas, oil, cumin, garlic, lemon and salt in the middle of the tray and mix thoroughly to coat the chickpeas in the seasoning. Spread out thinly and try to avoid them touching each other as much as possible.

Roast on the highest shelf in the oven for 15–20 minutes, until they're a little tanned, quite crunchy and dry on the outside, and still a little soft on the inside. Give them a stir halfway through the cooking time.

Remove from the oven and immediately scatter the parsley and the chilli flakes over, mixing to coat, then transfer the chickpeas and any loose parsley to a storage container and let it cool (without closing the lid). Store leftovers in the fridge.

TO ASSEMBLE
Per Bento

1 portion of pre-prepped
  sweet gratitude rice
  (page 37)
a small handful of dandelion
  greens
a small handful of salad greens
¼ avocado, flesh scooped out
  or in chunks
1 tbsp tamari seeds (page 44)
1 wedge of lime
a scatter of goji berries or
  sultanas, rinsed briefly under
  the tap, optional

Arrange the rice in one end of your box, and mix the dandelion and salad greens together in the other end of the box. Push the leaves to the edge and pile the avocado and seeds on top (this is your 'dry dressing'). In the remaining space, add the chick'n peas and lime, and finish with a scattering of goji berries. Close your box and pack in a bento bag or furoshiki with a fork or chopsticks.

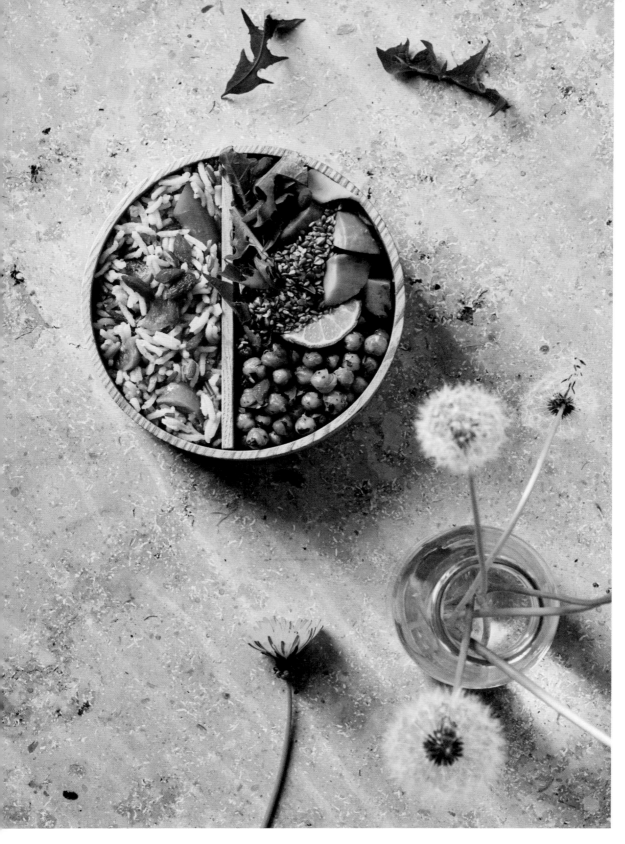

Summer in a Jar

___

When the weather is warm, this dish is great for lunch, and dinner too. The base is courgettes cut into ribbons – courgetti – and ripe summer tomatoes. Courgettes are natural blotters, great drenched in sauce, however when left in something salty (the sauce) they start juicing up, which is impractical for a bento. This is where my little trick comes in: mix the courgette and tomato sauce with a few chunks of stale sourdough (or a few scoops of quinoa), like a panzanella bread salad, and the courgette juice gets soaked up. Nothing is wasted, and you'll have a filling meal without even touching a pot or pan.

Makes 1 portion.
Fridge life: 24 hours.

Courgetti and Tomato Panzanella
2 large, ripe tomatoes
1 tbsp extra virgin olive oil
1 tsp coconut palm sugar
1 tsp balsamic vinegar
½ tsp Herbs de Provence
   or dried rosemary
1 tsp smoked paprika
½ tsp sea salt
black pepper, to taste
1 small courgette, cut into ribbons
1 slice of stale sourdough bread, or
   around 100g pre-prepped, cold quinoa
   (page 31)
a big handful of mixed salad greens,
   including some herbs like mint or basil,
   if possible

Optional add-ons:
½ red pepper, finely chopped
a handful of toasted almonds, roughly
   chopped
a scattering of olives or capers
1 spring onion, finely chopped

Use a leak-proof bento box or jar with a lid for this bento. Coarsely grate one of the tomatoes into a big mixing bowl (discard the skin), then add the rest of the panzanella ingredients (except the bread/quinoa), including the second tomato, chopped-up. Combine well until the courgette ribbons have softened a little, half a minute. Tear or break the bread into bite-sized pieces and gently toss with the courgette mixture (make sure you use a good artisan bread with a crust or you'll end up with a very mushy salad).

Transfer the panzanella into your jar or box and layer any add ons and salad greens on top. Close your container and pack in a bento bag or furoshiki with a fork or chopsticks.

TIP:
For a photogenic jar, like the image, don't mix the courgetti and tomatoes, and layer everything separately.

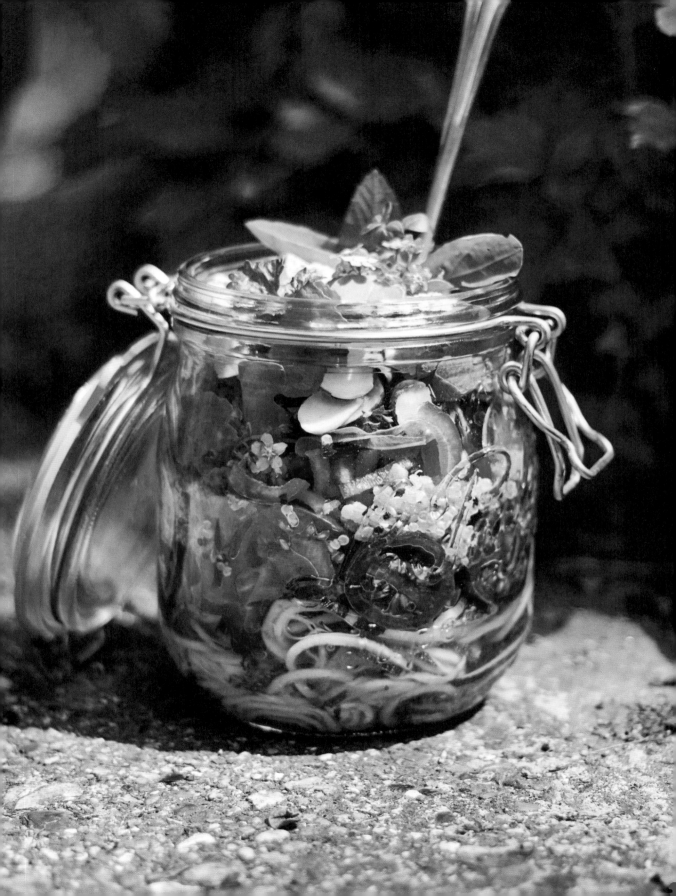

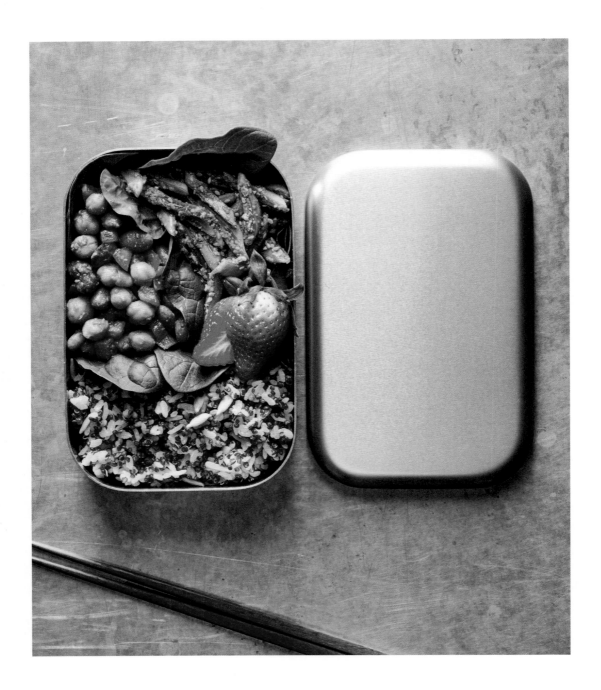

Double Act Bean Bento

There are plant proteins aplenty in this bento: quinoa-boosted rice, rich and smoky smashed miso beans and 'goma-ae', green beans in a classic Japanese crushed sesame marinade (made less classic by adding the beans raw not cooked!). Beans are something me and Andy sometimes grow in our London garden and a summer of many, many runner beans is how this dish came about. Raw goma-ae is just as good with other green beans too!

Makes 2 bento.
Fridge life: up to 24 hours.

Smashed smoky miso beans makes 2–4 portions. Fridge life: up to 3 days.

Raw goma-ae makes 2 portions.
Fridge life: up to 3 days.

Smashed Smoky Miso Beans

2 tbsp brown rice miso paste
½ tbsp brown rice vinegar
½ tbsp coconut palm sugar
1 tsp smoked paprika
1 tsp gochugaru (Korean red pepper) or ½ tsp chilli flakes
a little finely grated unwaxed lemon zest, optional
½ tsp garlic granules, optional
1 red pepper, finely diced
240g cooked mixed beans (drained and rinsed, if using canned)

Stir together all the ingredients, except the pepper and beans, to a paste, either in a mixing bowl or directly in a storage container (big enough to fit the beans as well). Add the red pepper and beans and combine well, 'smashing' the beans a little, either with a spoon, or, if using a storage container, by closing the lid and shaking hard. This is ready to eat straight away, but is best after marinating for a few hours (just in time for lunch!). Store leftovers in a (glass) storage container with a lid, in the fridge.

Raw Goma-ae

150g runner, flat or string beans
4 tbsp white or whole toasted sesame seeds (page 41), crushed (see Tip)
1 tbsp tamari
1 tsp brown rice vinegar

Wash, trim and cut the beans thinly (5mm) on the diagonal. Add them directly to a storage container with the rest of the goma-ae ingredients, and combine.

TO ASSEMBLE
Per Bento

1 portion of pre-prepped quinoa-sunflower rice (page 35)
a few large salad leaves
1 strawberry, optional

Arrange the rice in one end of your box. Use the salad leaves as separators, or bowls, for the two types of beans in the remaining space. Finish with the strawberry, if using. Close your box and pack in a bento bag or furoshiki with a fork or chopsticks.

TIP:

If you don't have a pestle and mortar, crush the sesame seeds on your chopping board by firmly rolling the base of a clean glass jar over them a few times. Roughly crushed is fine.

Faux Smoked Salmon Scandi Bento

Mixing yesterday's rice with a quick-pickle is a great way to revive it. This one is inspired by my Scandinavian childhood's classic flavours. In the omelette, aonori seaweed adds a touch of the sea. If you prefer a seed omelette, use the recipe on page 132, adding the aonori. Liquid smoke, a game-changing, natural seasoning, used to be reserved for chefs and food manufacturers but now it's easy to source from well-stocked supermarkets or online and will give your faux smoked salmon an authentic flavour.

Makes 1 bento.
Fridge life: up to 24 hours.

Faux salmon rice makes 2 portions.
Fridge life: up to 2 days.
Thin egg omelette makes 1 portion.
Fridge life: up to 2 days.

Faux Salmon Rice

½ medium carrot, coarsely grated
  (see Tip)
1 tsp brown rice vinegar
1 tsp maple syrup or clear honey
½ tsp liquid smoke seasoning
  or ½ tsp smoked paprika
1 tbsp flaxseed oil
a few dill fronds or leaves, torn
  or ½ tsp dried dill
½ tsp sea salt
freshly ground black pepper, to taste
2 portions of pre-prepped brown short-
  grain rice, about 1 batch (page 30)

In the evening, combine the carrot with the rest of the faux salmon rice ingredients, except for the rice, in a mixing bowl. Cover and leave to marinate overnight, or for at least 2 hours. In the morning, add the rice to the marinated mix and combine well. (Store leftovers in an airtight container in the fridge.)

Thin Omelette

1 large organic egg
½ tsp tamari
1 tsp aonori seaweed or a small sprig of
  parsley, finely chopped
black pepper, to taste
a little oil, to fry

Add all the omelette ingredients, except for the oil for frying, to a big glass jar with a lid, screw the lid on tight and give it a really good shake. Heat a frying pan over a medium heat, rub with a little oil and pour all the batter in, tilting your pan to get a crêpe. When its surface starts looking matte, gently flip over and cook for another few seconds. Fold the thin omelette in three, transfer to a clean chopping board and cut crossways into fine shreds.

TO ASSEMBLE

a few little gem lettuce leaves
1–2 tbsp sauerkraut, juice
  drained off
½ apple, cut into chunks
¼ avocado, flesh scooped out
  or sliced
a few dill fronds to garnish,
  optional

Arrange the rice in one end of your box, and make a bed of salad leaves in the remaining space. Arrange the omelette, sauerkraut, apple and avocado on top of the leaves and finish with a little black pepper and fresh dill, if using. Close your box and pack in a bento bag or furoshiki with a fork or chopsticks.

TIP:
To get the beautifully shaped strands of carrot as in the image, use a julienne mandolin.

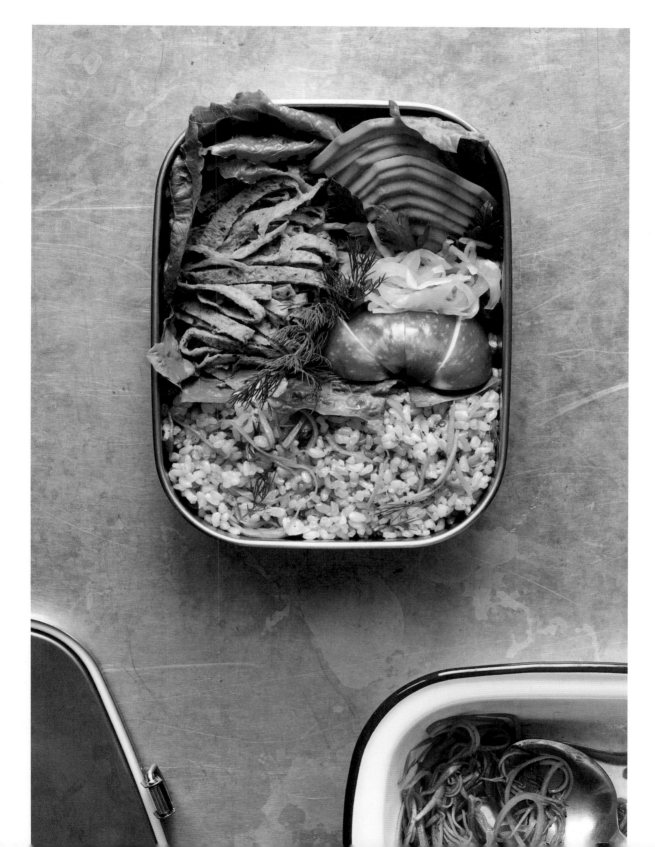

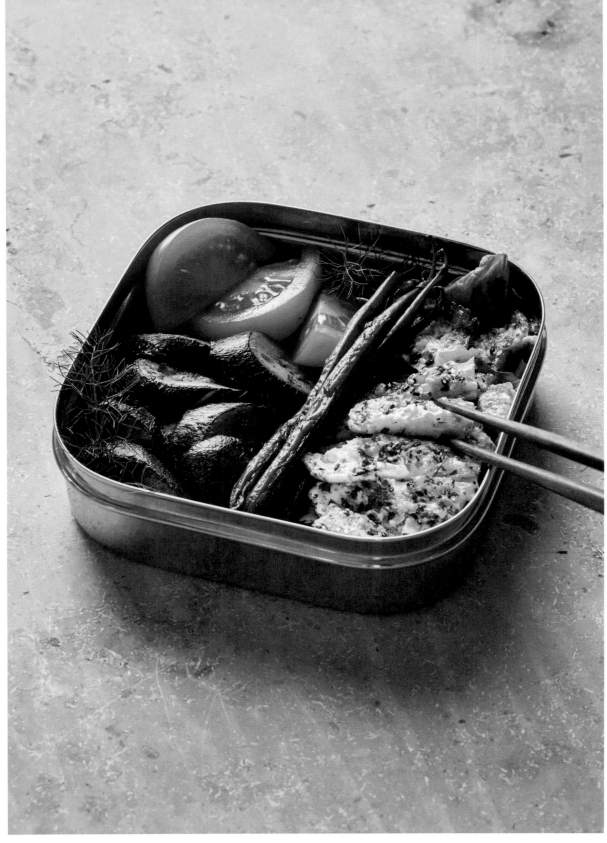

Grandmother's Dill Courgette Bento

My Bulgarian grandmother taught me how to make almost all of her classic dishes. She would sit on her chair in her kitchen, instructing me what to do, making sure I took notes (oh I treasure those!). This is based on one of those dishes: diagonally cut courgette discs, stacked like fallen dominos and roasted in the oven. Mine are made bento-time-friendly, in a pan on the stove. This recipe is without grains (but you can add some if you like).

Makes 1 bento.
Fridge life: 24 hours.

Pan-seared-steamed Dill Courgette

1 small-medium courgette, cut into thick (2cm) discs on the diagonal
1 small handful of green beans, washed but not trimmed
50–100ml water (depends on the size of your pan)
1 tbsp tamari
½ tsp chilli flakes
½ tsp dried dill (see Tip)
black pepper, to taste
1 pinch of garlic granules, optional

Heat a dry medium frying pan to very hot (a cast iron pan is ideal, but a normal pan will also work), and pour the water, tamari, and the rest of the seasonings into a glass. Lay the courgette discs out side by side in the hot pan, making sure they don't overlap, but are touching the surface fully. Place the beans wherever there's space (less important that they touch the surface fully). Use a spatula, or lay a second, clean frying pan to press down on the courgettes from the top, giving them a slight char (2–3 minutes). Flip the discs over and press for another minute or so (make sure the beans don't burn), then, have a big lid or heatproof plate ready, and pour all the seasoned water over the veggies and quickly cover the pan with the lid.

Allow to steam over a medium heat, until all the water has evaporated and the courgettes are tender but not soggy (2–3 minutes). Add more water if it looks like it needs a little more time. Tip the veggies out on a plate to cool, then give the pan a brief rinse before making the herb-fried egg.

Herb-fried egg

a little oil, to fry
1 medium or large organic egg
1 tsp sesame seeds (any type, not toasted)
a handful of finely chopped parsley
sea salt and chilli flakes, to taste

Heat the frying pan over a medium heat. Add a little oil and scatter half of the sesame seeds into the oil to fizzle for a few seconds, then crack the egg on top. Scatter the rest of the seeds, parsley and salt on the egg. For speed, you can pop the yolk (avoid runny eggs for bento food safety). When the yolk seems firm, flip and fry for a few more moments then slide onto a chopping board and cut into bite-sized strips (easier to pick out of the box). Let it cool slightly before packing in your bento box.

TO ASSEMBLE
Per Bento

1 large, ripe tomato
a few salad leaves
fresh herbs, to garnish, optional

Cut the tomato into large pieces and add in one end of your bento box, then add the courgette and beans, stacked up snug close to the tomato. Use the lettuce to line the remaining space in the box, and place your egg slices on top. Garnish with herbs if using. Close your box and pack in a bento bag or furoshiki with a fork or chopsticks.

TIP:

You can use Herbes de Provence or dried rosemary instead of dill.

Tofu Steak Boost Bento

If you haven't tried freezing your tofu before cooking it, now is the time! Everything that can be a little boring about tofu; 'bland', 'wobbly', 'meh' is swopped for an airier, drier structure that soaks up seasoning and gets a good crust when fried. Different brands of tofu come out slightly differently, but go for a soft to medium type that comes in liquid in a small box (silken or very firm tofu won't work) and pop it in your freezer without opening the packet until frozen solid, then thaw completely. Add a lick of spice, mineral-rich, mixed-grain rice and gomashio (sesame salt) and you have a real power bento right here!

TIP:
Tofu steaks are yummy cut into chunks and used in any recipes in this book that call for smoked tofu. The chunks soak up flavour really well.

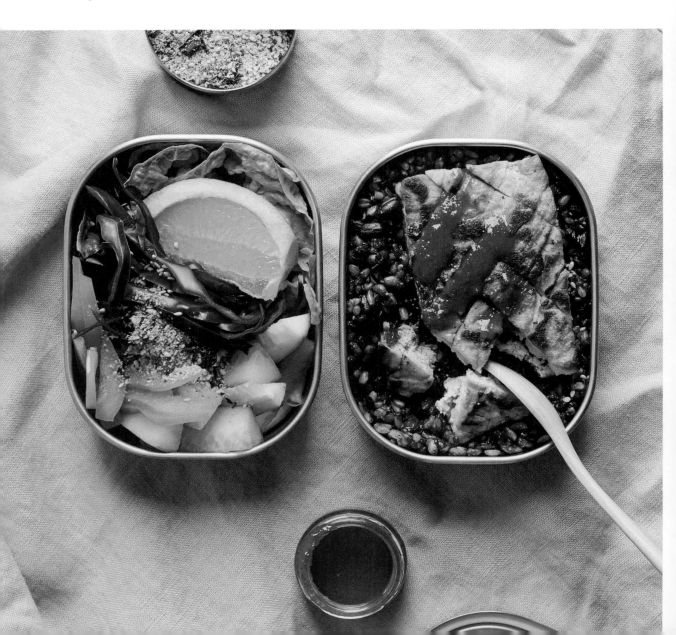

Makes 1 bento.

Makes 4 tofu steaks.
Fridge life: up to 4 days.

Tofu Steaks

1 x 400g block of tofu, frozen once,
  then thawed
2 tbsp tamari or 1½ tbsp fish sauce
  (vegetarian)
about 4cm piece fresh ginger,
  finely grated
a little oil, to fry

Remove the thawed tofu block from its
packaging and give it a brief squeeze
between your palms over the sink to
drain off some liquid. Cut the block into
4 steaks, then score each one deeply in
a cross pattern to absorb the seasonings
better. Leave the steaks on your chopping
board and drizzle the tamari or fish sauce
over and hand-squeeze the grated ginger
to extract its juice (discard the pulp).

Give the steaks a couple of pushes from
the top to absorb the juicy seasonings
(like sponges!).

TIP:
Water used for quick-blanching
veggies can, once cooled,
be used to water your house
plants. As long as no salt,
seasonings or oils are added,
all cooking water can be used
like this and your plants will
love you for the extra nutrients!
Leftover, pure coffee and tea
can be used the same way.

Preheat a frying pan until very hot, then
add the oil and the tofu steaks. Press down
on the steaks with a spatula to char the
underside (do the same for the other side
when you flip them over) and fry for 2–4
minutes on each side. Transfer to a plate
and leave to cool. (Store leftovers in an
airtight container in the fridge.)

Quick-blanched Red Cabbage

1–2cm wedge of red cabbage, thinly
  shredded
½ tsp maple or agave syrup
1 tsp apple cider vinegar
a pinch of sea salt

To quick-blanch the red cabbage, place
it in a heatproof bowl and pour boiling
water over to submerge. Leave for
5 minutes (and marvel at the deep blue
water – see Tip) then drain in a strainer
and cool completely under a cold running
tap, tip onto a paper towel and briefly pat
dry. Return the cabbage to your chopping
board and toss with the syrup, vinegar
and salt using your hands.

TO ASSEMBLE

1 portion of pre-prepped multi-
  multi rice (page 35)
cheatin' gochujang sauce or
  Korean-style dressing, to taste
  (pages 48 and 47)
a few leaves of little gem lettuce,
  shredded
5cm cucumber, cut into thick sticks
¼ pepper, thinly sliced
1 wedge of orange
2–3 tbsp dulse gomashio or any
  gomashio (page 41)

Arrange the rice in one end of
your bento box (or in a whole
box, if using a double-decker
like in the image) and top with
1 or 2 tofu steaks. Season with
gochujang or dressing, or pack
the liquid in a separate small
container to take with you.

Make a bed of lettuce in the other
end of the box (or the second
double-decker box). Arrange the
red cabbage, cucumber, pepper
and orange on top and scoop
a few generous spoonfuls of
gomashio over the veggies.

Once it's time to eat, you can
squeeze the orange over for a
make-shift dressing (it will merge
with the gomashio). Close your
box and pack in a bento bag or
furoshiki with a fork or chopsticks.

Golden Roast Squash Bento

It's hard not to love roast squash, especially with this kind of colour! My favourite is Crown Prince (pictured), which has dense and quite dry flesh. I like making the most of my oven's heat by leaving the roast in for a while after turning the heat off. Each oven is different though, so use my timings as a guide. 'Su-no-mono' translates as 'vinegar thing' – a classic, tangy-sweet cucumber and seaweed salad. Here's my simplified and (quite) de-sugared version.

Makes 1 bento.
Fridge life: up to 24 hours.

Golden roast squash makes 4–5 portions.
Fridge life: up to 5 days.
Su-no-mono makes 2 portions.
Fridge life: up to 2 days.
Cabbage quick-pickle makes 2–3 portions.
Fridge life: up to 1 week.

Golden Roast Squash

1kg squash
2 tbsp extra virgin olive oil
1 tsp sea salt

Preheat the oven to 220°C /425°F/gas mark 7 and line a large baking tray with baking paper.

Peel, if needed, and de-seed your squash and cut into large (3–4cm) chunks. Cutting slightly irregular triangle-shapes means they'll cook faster, while still being chunky, and each piece will feel a little different in your mouth. Pile the pieces onto your baking sheet and thoroughly coat in oil and salt using your hands. Roast on the highest shelf in the oven for 20 minutes. Turn the oven off and leave the squash to finish cooking in the residual heat for 10 minutes. Remove from the heat and let it cool slightly before packing in a bento. (Store leftovers in an airtight container in the fridge.)

Su-no-mono

½ tbsp instant dried wakame seaweed
8cm (100g) cucumber
½ tsp sea salt
2cm piece fresh ginger, finely grated
1½ tbsp brown rice vinegar
1 tsp agave syrup
a pinch of gochugaru (Korean pepper), optional

Rehydrate the wakame in a bowl of plenty of cold water for 10 minutes (it will expand 4–5 times), then drain and squeeze out as much water as you can with your hands. Chop roughly.

Thinly slice the cucumber (1–2mm), using a mandolin if you have one, and add it and the salt to a colander sitting over your sink and gently mix with your hands until the cucumber starts sweating, about 30 seconds. Leave it to drip while the wakame rehydrates, then rinse the salt off and gently squeeze as much liquid out as possible without breaking the slices.

Add the cucumber and the rehydrated wakame to a small storage container and squeeze the ginger over (discard the pulp), then add the rest of the ingredients and mix well. Store leftovers in the fridge.

Simplest Cabbage Quick-pickle

100g red or white cabbage, very thinly sliced (use a mandolin if you have one)
2 tbsp apple cider vinegar
1 tsp sea salt

Add all ingredients to a sturdy plastic bag or small bowl, then follow the instructions for purple quick-pickle on page 139.

TO ASSEMBLE

1 portion brown short-grain rice (page 30) – the rice in the image was cooked with a handful of small, dried green soy beans
a handful of mixed salad greens
½ small chioggia beetroot, very thinly sliced
1–2 tbsp savoury granola (page 43)
pink peppercorns, to taste, optional

Arrange the rice in one end of your box and make a bed of salad greens in the remaining space. Arrange the squash, su-no-mono and cabbage in separate mounds on top of the leaves and finish with a small mound of savoury granola and some pink peppercorns, if using. Close your box and pack in a bento bag or furoshiki with a fork or chopsticks.

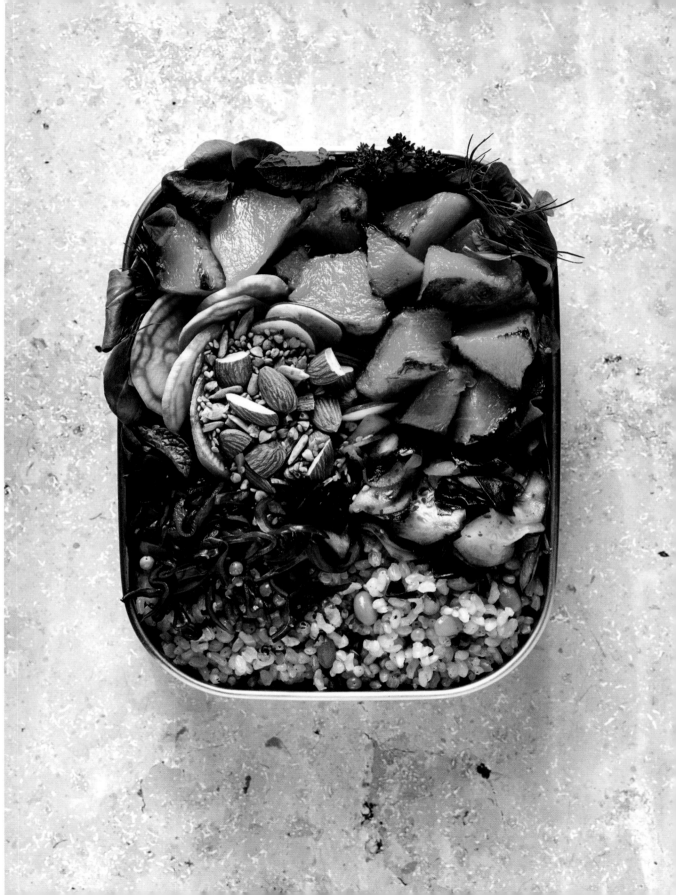

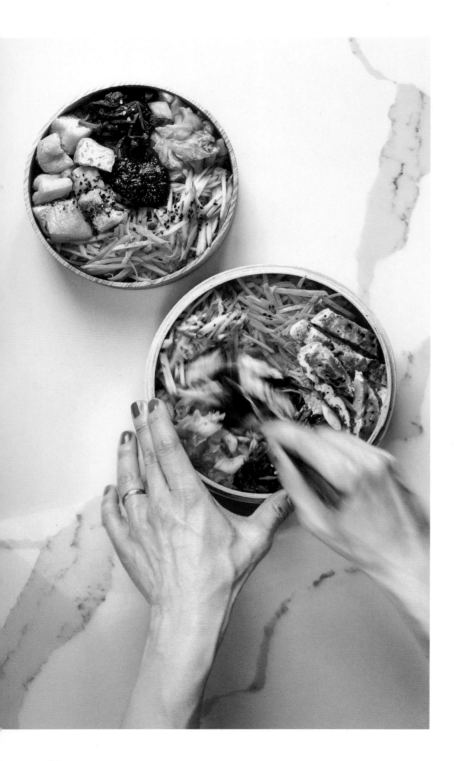

TIP:
The gochujang makes enough
for 4–6 bentos. It's very
versatile: Mix a little with
raw, sliced cucumber, carrot
or cabbage for an instant
quick-pickle. Dilute with a little
water for a salad dressing. Mix
with nut butter or tahini for a
delicious spread or dip. Toss
with vegetables and a little oil
for oven-roasting.

Cheatin' Bibimbap Bento

The Korean national dish bibimbap can be pretty addictive! Cheatin'
Bibimbap is my fast fix, without any ready-made ingredients – and
without garlic so I can indulge at any time of the day (although you are
welcome to add some garlic if you like!). The essentials of kimchi and
gochujang sauce can both be tricky to source and time-consuming to
make, but my cheating versions are ready in minutes.

Makes 1 bento, with kimchi and
gochujang to spare

Cheatin' Gochujang Sauce

Prepare one batch, page 48.

Cheatin' Kimchi

250g Chinese cabbage (about ¼
   medium), cut lengthways in 3cm strips,
   then in bite-sized chunks (3–4cm)
1 tsp sea salt
4cm piece fresh ginger, finely minced
1 spring onion, finely sliced on the
   diagonal
1 tbsp gochugaru (Korean pepper),
   see Tip
2 tsp fish sauce (vegetarian)
½ tsp agave syrup

Place the cabbage in a strainer over
your sink, sprinkle the salt over then
massage with your hands until the
cabbage starts to soften and release
a little liquid, about 1 minute. Leave in
the strainer while you prepare the spice
mix: add the remaining ingredients to a
mixing bowl and use a spatula or big
spoon to mix, pressing on the ginger and
spring onion to soften them a little.

Rinse the salt off the cabbage and
squeeze it in your hands to remove as
much liquid as possible. Add it to the
spice mix and combine well. Transfer to
a glass jar with a lid.

What you don't use straight away, leave
out for 24–48 hours before refrigerating:
this will start a slight fermentation which
adds both to the flavour and to your
gut happiness.

TIP:
Substitute the gochugaru with 1
tsp chilli flakes, 1 tsp paprika
and 1 tsp sweet smoked
paprika, combined.

TO ASSEMBLE

50g (big handful) baby spinach
½ medium carrot, julienned
   or grated
⅓ cucumber, julienned or sliced
1 portion of white Japanese or
   brown short-grain rice (pages
   29 and 30)
1 egg, fried then cut into bite-
   sized strips (make sure the
   yolk is well done) or 1 portion
   pre-fried tofu cubes
½ tsp brown rice vinegar
½ tsp toasted sesame oil
½ tsp tamari
toasted sesame seeds, to taste
1 spring onion, finely sliced

Pour boiling water over the
spinach in a bowl, cover and
leave for 2 minutes. Cool under
the tap and squeeze with your
hands to remove as much water
as possible.

Make a bed of rice in your box.
Arrange the kimchi, spinach,
carrot, cucumber and egg or
tofu in small separate mounds
on top. Pour a little vinegar
and oil on the carrot and
cucumber, and a little tamari
on the spinach. Put a generous
tablespoon of the gochujang
in the middle and sprinkle with
toasted sesame seeds and
spring onion. To eat the Korean
way, stir everything together,
allowing the gochujang sauce
to flavour everything.

Iron Power and Goma-ae Bento

Here's another mineral-boosting bento! (Love them.) Brown rice, aduki, beetroot and raw cacao in the sister power rice, hijiki seaweed in the iron power salad and sesame in goma-ae beans are all mineral stars. The salad is based on the typical Japanese dish 'Hijiki-no-nimono', but I've reduced the steps, amount of sugar and intensity of cooking to get a Shiso-approved dish! Same for the goma-ae beans – less cooking and more of the good stuff (ie. pile that sesame high). Remember to bring a fruit rich in vitamin C as it helps your body to absorb the iron this bento is so rich in.

Makes 1 bento.
Fridge life: up to 24 hours.

Iron power salad makes 2–3 portions. Fridge life: up to a week.

Goma-ae beans makes 2–3 portions. Fridge life: up to 4 days.

Iron Power Salad

5g dried hijiki seaweed
  (about 1½ tbsp if crumbled)
½ tbsp coconut palm sugar
1 tbsp tamari
½ tbsp brown rice vinegar
about 2cm piece fresh ginger, finely grated and juice hand-squeezed straight into the cooking pan (pulp discarded)
1 large carrot (100g), peeled and cut into matchsticks

Place the hijiki in a bowl, crumbling it if the strands are quite long, then cover with plenty of cold water (it will expand 3–4 times) and leave to rehydrate for 15 minutes, then drain.

Add the seaweed and the remaining iron power salad ingredients, except the carrots, to a small pan. Simmer over a low heat, stirring occasionally, until just a little liquid remains, 5–10 minutes. Remove from the heat, add the carrots and combine. Let it cool and transfer to a glass storage container with a lid and store in the fridge. It's ready to eat straight away, but is best after marinating for a few hours (just in time for lunch!).

Goma-ae Beans

100g green beans
4 tbsp toasted sesame seeds (page 41)
1 tbsp tamari
½ tbsp brown rice vinegar

Quick-blanch the green beans by placing them whole in a heatproof bowl and pouring boiling water over to submerge. Leave for 5 minutes, then drain in a strainer and cool completely under a cold running tap. Remove their woody ends (but keep the tails on as they're cute!) and cut into 3cm lengths. Crush the sesame seeds either in a pestle and mortar (See Tip) or a small blender, taking care not to over-blend. Combine the beans with the rest of the Goma-ae ingredients directly in a storage container. Again, this is ready to eat straight away, but is best after the beans have been marinating for a few hours.

Variation:
Instead of green beans, use ⅓ head of broccoli, florets quartered.

TO ASSEMBLE

1 portion of pre-prepped sister power rice (page 37)
a few little gem lettuce leaves
a few drops of toasted sesame oil and a pinch of sea salt
1 overnight egg (page 51), halved, and/or a handful of saltwater-toasted nuts and seeds (page 44)
1 satsuma, or other citrus fruit

Arrange the rice in one end of your box and use the lettuce leaves as separators between the rice, the salad and the beans. Wedge your egg in, if using, topping it with a little oil and salt, and finish with a handful of nuts in a small mound. Close your box and pack, along with the satsuma, in a bento bag or furoshiki with a fork or chopsticks.

TIP:

If you don't have a pestle and mortar, crush the sesame seeds on your chopping board by firmly rolling the base of a clean glass jar over them a few times. Roughly crushed is fine.

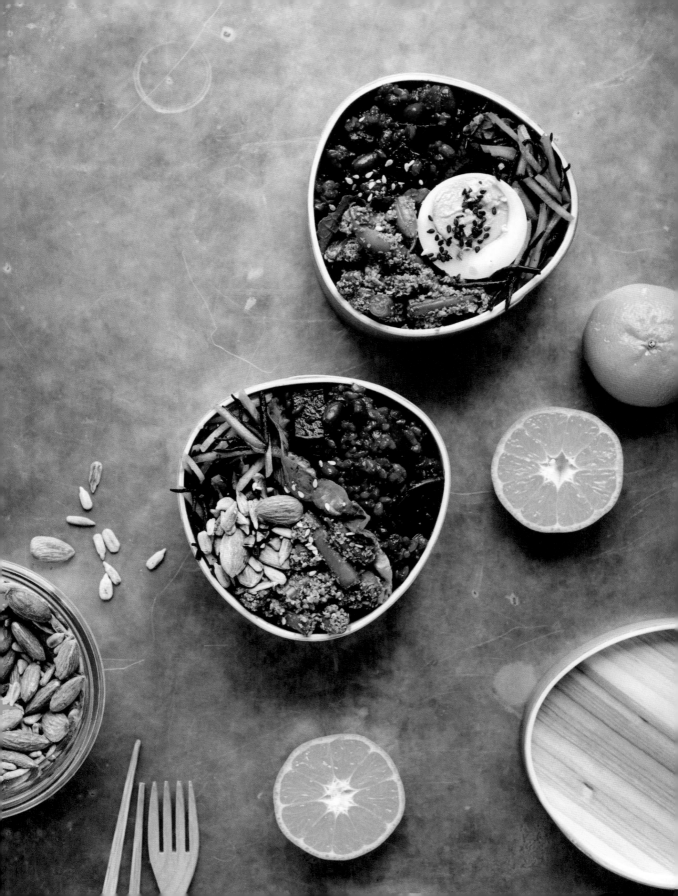

Roast Cabbage Slaw Bento

I almost accidentally discovered how good cabbage is roasted. I'd been looking at 'grilled cabbage' recipes online but they were all for big wedges of cabbage (which seemed too time-consuming for an everyday recipe). Instead, I sliced my cabbage really thin, like a slaw, and roasted it spread thinly over a large baking tray. Since that moment it's on repeat in our house! The heat changes the cabbage into something much sweeter and full of umami, and the small pieces of lemon add a surprise aromatic burst to every few bites. I started adding in cooked chickpeas or tofu too, to make it into a simple weekday meal (amazing wedged with avocado in a tortilla too) and since it's so easy to make and tastes good cold, it's great for bento too.

Roast cabbage slaw
makes 3–4 portions.
Fridge life: up to
4 days.

Roast Cabbage Slaw

½ medium (about 300g) red cabbage,
    finely shredded
240g cooked chickpeas (drained and
    rinsed, if using canned)
1 small, tart apple, coarsely grated
2 tbsp extra virgin olive oil
finely grated zest and juice of
    ½ unwaxed lemon
1 wedge of that same lemon, cut across
    into 3mm slices
1 tsp sea salt
½ tsp dried chilli flakes
¼ tsp fennel seeds and/or cumin seeds
½ tsp garlic granules, optional

Preheat the oven to 220°C/425°F/ gas mark 7. Line a large baking tray with baking paper. Use a big, open tray rather than a high-edged tray or casserole.

Pile all the ingredients in the middle of the tray and combine with your hands, then spread thinly – you want the ingredients to be minimally overlapping, so they get a chance to dehydrate a little. Roast at the highest shelf in the oven for 15–20 minutes, stirring once halfway through, until the cabbage is slightly charred at the edges and the chickpeas have a little tan.

Remove from heat and leave to cool slightly, then use the existing baking paper to wrap around the mixture like a fish and chip packet. This keeps the moisture and flavour in, and saves washing up an oily storage container later. Once cool, store the packet in the fridge (in a bowl).

TO ASSEMBLE
Per Bento
Fridge life: up to 24 hours.

BENTO 1: Soba Noodle

1 portion (85g) dry soba
    noodles
⅓ batch roast cabbage slaw
2–3 little gem lettuce leaves
¼ avocado, flesh scooped out
    or sliced
2 tbsp gomashio (any type)
    or toasted sesame seeds
    (page 41)
blueberries, to taste

Cook the soba according to the packet's instructions. Drain in a colander, cool completely under a running cold tap, then let them drip-dry for a few minutes, or instantly spin-dry them in a sturdy salad spinner. Place the soba in your bento box. Push them to one side and add the lettuce and a portion of the cabbage slaw in the remaining space. Add the avocado and spoon a mound of gomashio onto the noodles. Finish with a scatter of blueberries. Close your box and pack in a bento bag or furoshiki with a fork or chopsticks.

Fridge life: eat the same day

BENTO 2: Onigirazu – 'Sushi Sandwich'

2 nori sheets
300g pre-prepped black
    gradient rice (page 34),
    see Tip
⅓ batch roast cabbage slaw
½ avocado, flesh scooped out
    or sliced
50g smoked tofu, in thin slices
    (Taifun brand is ideal), optional
blueberries, to taste

Follow the instructions on pages 130–131 for how to make the onigirazu, using the nori sheets, and topping the rice with a portion of the cabbage slaw, the avocado and tofu. Sliced avocado is easier to layer evenly in onigirazu. Pack in your bento box with a handful of blueberries. Close your box and pack in a bento bag or furoshiki with a napkin.

TIP:
To get the lilac rice tint in the image, cook black gradient rice according to instructions on page 34, but use 240g white rice and just 20g black rice.

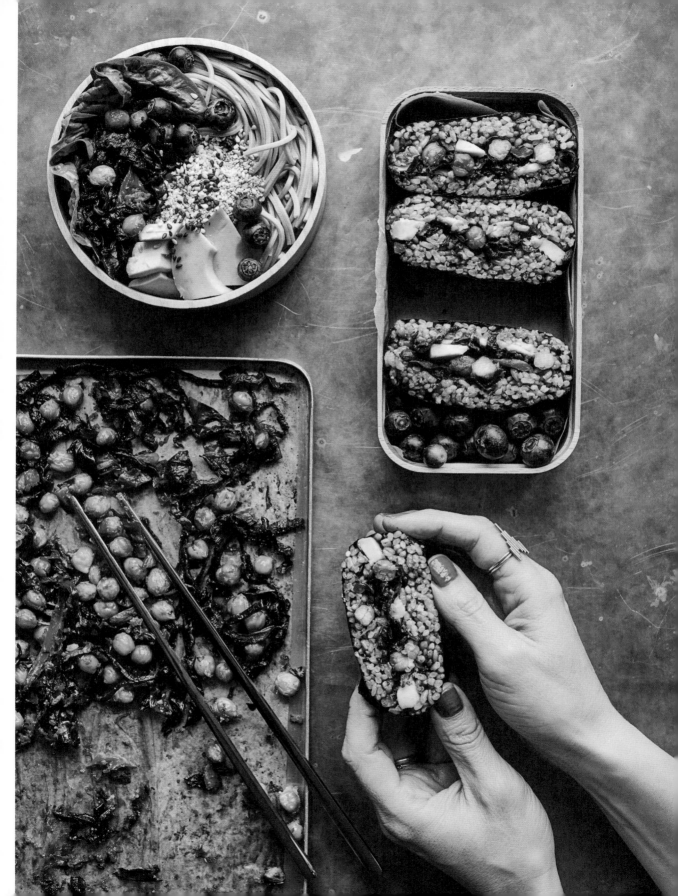

After the Show Bento – Tofu Sandwich Skewers and Tamago-yaki

I threw this together (okay, I'd already prepped the tamago-yaki!) to bring to a dear friend after her show at the theatre. I figured she would be ready for some power snacks after 1.5 hours of bouncing around stage (she was delighted! I just wished I'd brought more). The skewers may look complicated but there's a simple, fool-proof hack to make several in one go. Tamago-yaki is delicious cut chunky like this – especially good eaten speared with a cocktail stick. Both dishes make great canapés, too!

Makes 1 bento.
Fridge life: eat the same day

Tofu Sandwich Skewers

50g smoked, firm tofu (Viana brand is ideal, Taifun brand also works)
1 fig, thinly sliced (5mm), see Tip
5cm cucumber, thinly sliced (5mm)
5–6 fresh mint leaves
6–8 wooden cocktail sticks

Cut the tofu in thin (6–8mm) slices across, like you'd slice a loaf of bread. Now make a 'multi-store sandwich' (1) using the tofu slices as bread, and a single layer of fig or cucumber topped with mint leaf in between each. Make the layers as even as possible. When you've used up all the tofu slices and fillings, carefully spear the sandwich from the top (2), all the way to the bottom, with two neat rows of cocktail sticks (the number of sticks will depend on the size of your sandwich). Use a big, sharp knife to cut straight through the stack (3), between each stick. Voilà, tofu sandwich skewers!

TIP:
You can fill your sandwich skewers with anything that's not too wet or soft, I often make them with kiwi, pear, or pepper. The white flowers in the image are home-grown, edible borage.

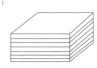

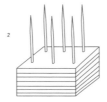

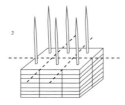

TO ASSEMBLE

a few salad leaves (I used pink radicchio)
1 portion tamago-yaki (page 134), cut into thick slices (3cm), each slice halved on the diagonal
½ red grapefruit, skin removed with a sharp knife, then sliced
a few raspberries

Use either one bento box or a few smaller containers to assemble. Line the bento box with the salad leaves and arrange the skewers and tamago on top, using leaves as separators if needed. The grapefruit is very juicy, so keep it separated from the tamago. Close the lid/s and pack in a bento bag or furoshiki with a napkin. To eat, you can use one of the sticks from the skewers to spear the tamago chunks.

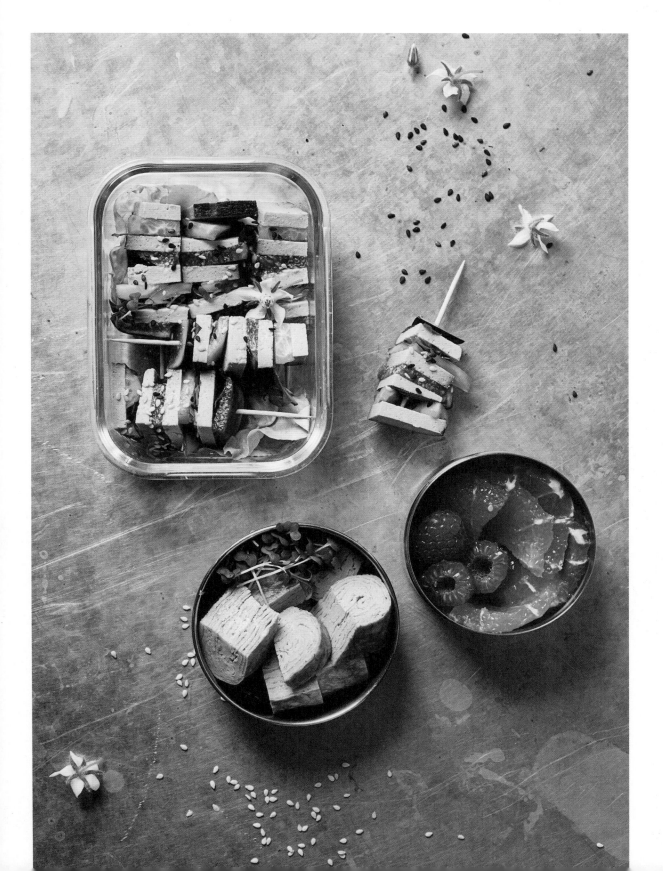

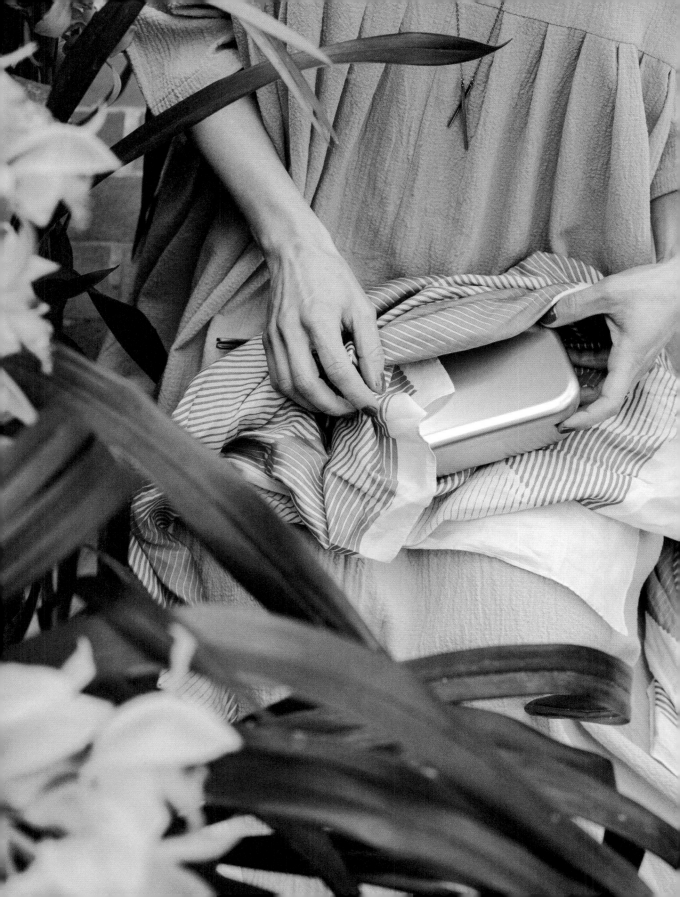

FANTASY BENTO

So much creative magic can happen within the
bounds of a box. Here are a dreamy handful of
gems from my bento journey to date.

Starry Sky Bento

It's all about the pink and green 'stars' in this beauty. The dark sky in this image is
a photographic background you may already have at home, a well-used cheap
metal baking tray. It's a brilliant prop for small set-ups like this one. I (mostly) like
ingredients to look natural in an image, and will often scatter/drop ingredients
(like the pomegranate seeds and peas here) onto the set, then fine tune by moving
pieces around (using my hands, or my thinnest chopsticks) until I feel it's balanced
but doesn't look too perfect.

Makes 1 bento.
Fridge life: up to 24 hours.

Noodles

½ nest (50–75g) dry flat rice noodles
½ tsp toasted sesame oil
1 tsp umesu or a pinch of sea salt

Rehydrate the rice noodles in the same
way as thin rice vermicelli (page 86),
but leave them to soak in the hot water
for longer, 10 minutes. Toss the noodles
with the oil and umesu or salt.

TO ASSEMBLE

3–4 leaves of little gem lettuce
½ avocado, peeled and
  thinly sliced
1 portion of su-no-mono
  (page 152)
a handful of frozen peas, thawed
  in a bowl of cold water for
  5 minutes
a handful of whole almonds,
  toasted and roughly chopped
a small bunch of basil leaves
a pinch of gochugaru (Korean
  red pepper)
white and red pomegranate
  seeds, to taste
2 wild strawberries, optional

Line your box with a piece of
roughly ripped baking paper,
letting it peek up around the
edges. Arrange your noodles
in one end of your box, and
line the rest of the space with
lettuce. Gently give your sliced
avocado half a push to fan
out and place it on top of the
lettuce leaves, and frame it
with the su-no-mono, peas and
almonds. Decorate with the
basil, gochugaru, pomegranate
seeds and wild strawberries.

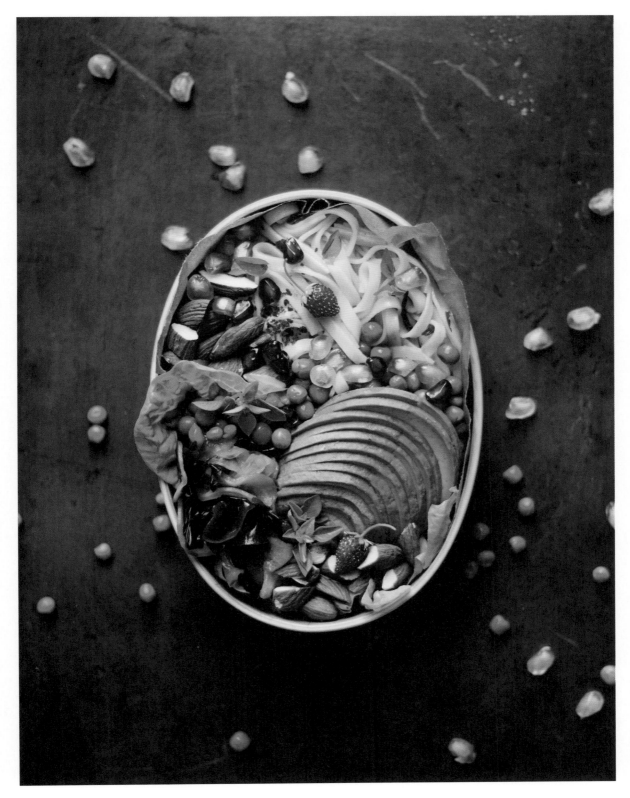

Fantasy Bento

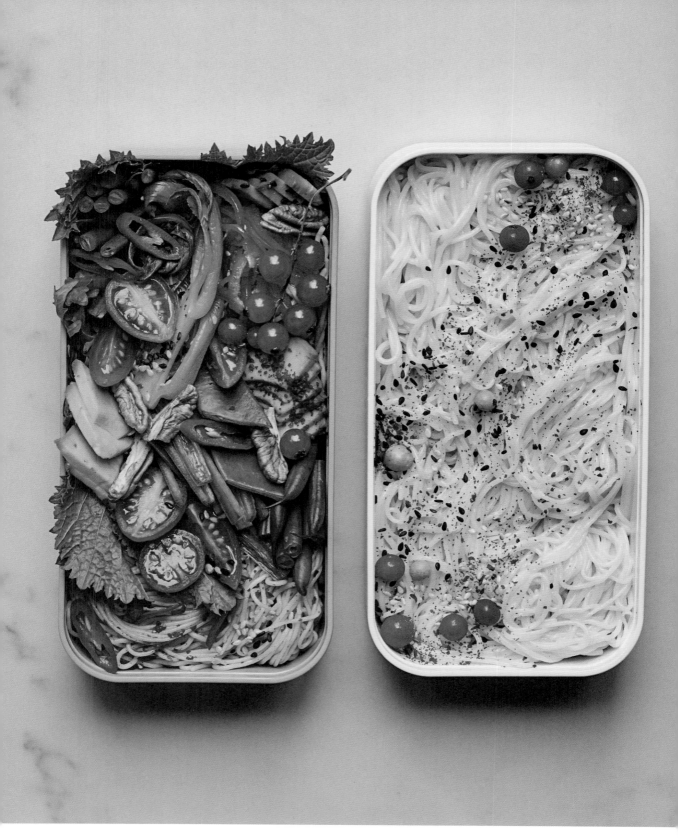

Snow White Bento

Snow White was one of my favourite tales as a kid, not the classic animation but the original Brothers Grimm's version. To me, it was clear she was the ONLY princess who was not blond, but explicitly with 'ebony hair, skin white as snow and lips red like blood'. There's something very powerful about these three colours and I've used them for as long as I can remember, whether in kids drawings, art installations or food!

When currants and wild strawberries are in season I freeze them in clusters to save for food styling – good quality, small-scale produced ones (or home-grown) will always look great and almost like fresh when thawed, like these in the image (and could you tell that the wild strawberries in the image on page 165 had been frozen too?).

Makes 1 bento.
Eat the same day.

1 nest (100g) dry rice vermicelli
1 tablespoon Korean style dressing (page 47)
1 bunch tatsoi greens, or a few chard leaves
a small handful of green beans
a small handful of mangetout
a small bunch of mustard greens, or other unusual-looking salad greens
¼ red romano pepper, very thinly sliced
¼ avocado, sliced
½ fresh large red chilli, thinly sliced on the diagonal
2–3 pecans
3 cherry tomatoes, halved
1 bunch of redcurrants
white and black toasted sesame seeds (page 41)
a few pinches of gochugaru (Korean red pepper)
sea salt, to taste

Use a double-decker box for this bento. Rehydrate, cool and drain the rice vermicelli (page 86). Separate a third out (use scissors to cut) and toss it with the Korean style dressing. Leave the rest of the noodles as they are.

Quick-blanch and cool the tatsoi, whole beans and whole mangetout. Wait to cut the veggies until after blanching – this makes the cuts look neater and stops them from 'bleeding' nutrients into the hot water. Cut the tatsoi in half lengthways, and then, depending on how big it is, save its prettiest part to be shown on top, and cut the rest into bite-sized pieces. Cut the mangetout on the diagonal and beans bunched up in 4–5cm pieces.

Push the red noodles up against the end of one box (they should fill about half of the box) and fill the second box evenly with the white noodles.

In the red noodle box, use the mustard leaves to make a 'frame' around the edges of the empty part of the box. Within this frame, arrange all your beautiful 'paints'. I tend to start with longer, more structured shapes (beans, leaves), then round shapes and finally tiny shapes, like cut chilli and sesame seeds.

To make the noodle box, simply scatter the noodles with sesame seeds, gochugaru, salt and a few redcurrants.

Green Matcha and Shiso Balls Bento

Two of my top magic ingredients in one ball: matcha green tea and shiso leaves. Something I always loved in Japan are foods delicately presented in leaves, as an edible way of appreciating the changing beauty of the seasons. A cherry tree leaf may envelop a sweet rice ball in spring, or a red acer leaf top a savoury treat in autumn. Shiso leaves are pretty rare to come by here in the UK, but you can, like myself, easily grow them in your garden (they are resilient to pests and love the climate here as far as I can tell!), or find them in speciality green grocers or Asian supermarkets. This is green shiso, see page 173 for red shiso leaves.

Makes 2 bento.

Makes 8 x 5–6cm diameter rice balls,
2 portions.
Fridge life: up to 24 hours.

1 batch of white Japanese rice (page 29)
8 green shiso leaves, stalks snipped off
    near the leaf
½ tsp matcha powder (ceremonial-grade
    gives the best vibrant colour)
½ tsp maple or agave syrup
½ tsp brown rice vinegar
a little water, to shape the balls
sea salt, to shape the balls
a sprinkle of toasted black sesame seeds
    (page 41), to decorate

Use freshly cooked rice, just cooled down to room temperature, or slightly warm (hot rice will discolour the shiso leaves). Part the rice into two halves. Stir the matcha, syrup and vinegar together to a paste in the bottom of a mixing bowl and add one half of the rice to the bowl. Gently mix through to colour the rice, taking care not to crush the grains too much.

Part the white and green halves in 4 each (you will have a total of 8 parts). Have a small bowl of cold water and sea salt ready. Wet your clean hands in the bowl, dab some sea salt on your palms (don't be stingy with the salt, as it both flavours and acts as a preservative for the rice balls) and shape each part of rice into a small ball. Wrap each ball in a shiso leaf. Wet and re-salt your hands between each.

Arrange the balls in your bento box, alternating green and white, and sprinkle the white balls with a little black sesame.

TIP
The balls are pretty filling by themselves, but you may want to bring a small container of toasted nuts and seeds (pages 43–44), or an unpeeled overnight egg (page 51) with you as well for extra power.

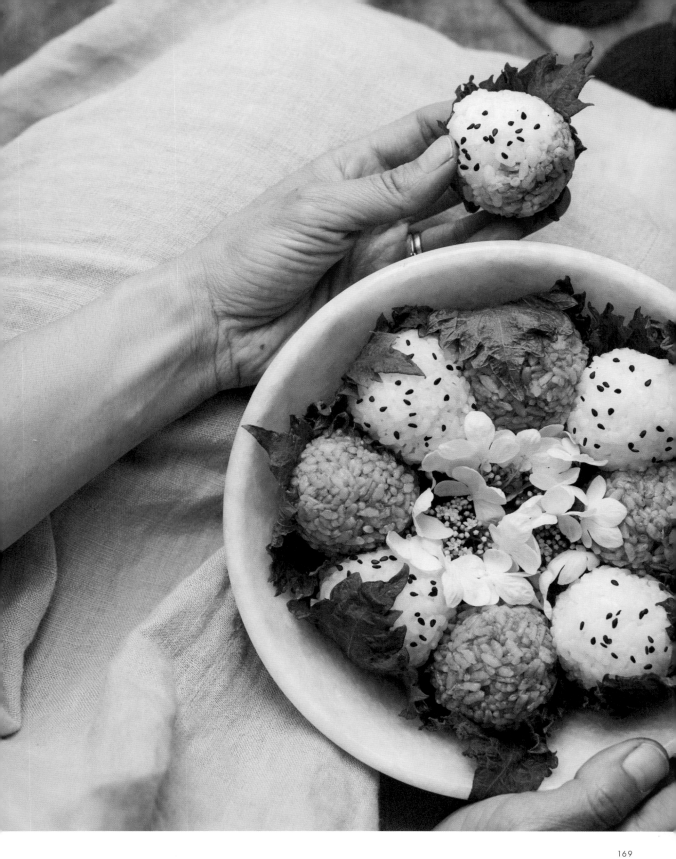

Fantasy Bento

Fairy Jewel Box Bento

_____

This bento has nearly broken the internet a few times! It could be the insanely pretty pink pomegranate jewels and white strawberries (aka pine berries) which I can only get hold of a few times a year. Or maybe the trick of colouring part of the noodles with beetroot and adding strands of green 'courgetti', as well as cutting everyday veggies in a party kind of way – mini cucumbers look completely new with a lengthways slice for example. If you have a 'melon baller' tool it can be used for any soft fruit and veg – here I've used it to make fun little avocado and kiwi balls.

Makes 1 portion.
Fridge life: up to 24 hours.

Quick-pickle Pink Cabbage

a tiny pinch of beetroot powder or a little
    grated raw beetroot
a pinch of sea salt
2 tbsp finely sliced white cabbage
½ tsp rice vinegar

Rub a tiny amount of beetroot powder or grated raw beetroot and the salt into the cabbage. You can work directly on your cutting board if you like. Add the vinegar and mix with your hands.

3-tone Noodles

½ nest of dry, thin rice vermicelli,
    rehydrated (page 86)
a tiny pinch of beetroot powder, or
    ¼ tsp grated raw beetroot + a squeeze
    of lemon
1 small courgette, ribboned with a fine-
    toothed julienne peeler, use a potato
    peeler for a wider 'cougettiatelle' look

Part the rice noodles half-half. Colour one half either by dabbing a tiny amount of beetroot powder into them, then gently mix with your hands to even the colour out, or add the grated beetroot into a glass, add ½ teaspoon water and a squeeze of lemon, then mix well with one noodle half.

Carefully dab a little salt into the courgetti strands to soften them slightly.

TO ASSEMBLE

a few little gem lettuce leaves
1 kiwi
½ avocado
1 mini cucumber
handful of mangetout, immersed
    in hot water for 2 minutes then
    rinsed cold
seeds from ¼ white pomegranate
    pine berries or small strawberries
amaranth sprouts

Using your hands or chopsticks, layer the noodles and courgetti, one type at a time, in a few layers. For the veg box, start with a bed of lettuce leaves, allowing some to peek out at the short edges of the box. Pile the cabbage in the middle of the box. Slice the blanched mangetout lengthways to show its seeds and arrange. Either mandolin or very thinly slice the cucumber lengthways and arrange in the box. Use a melon baller to make the avocado and kiwi balls, or slice as you wish using a very sharp knife, and arrange. Scatter the jewels over both boxes. Get your camera out, find some good light in front of your window and enjoy the magic.

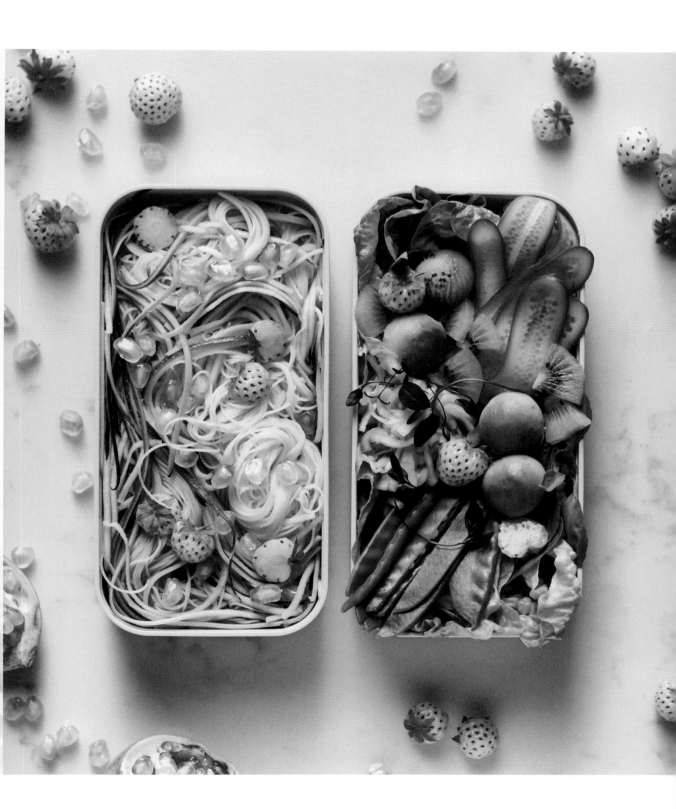

Fantasy Bento

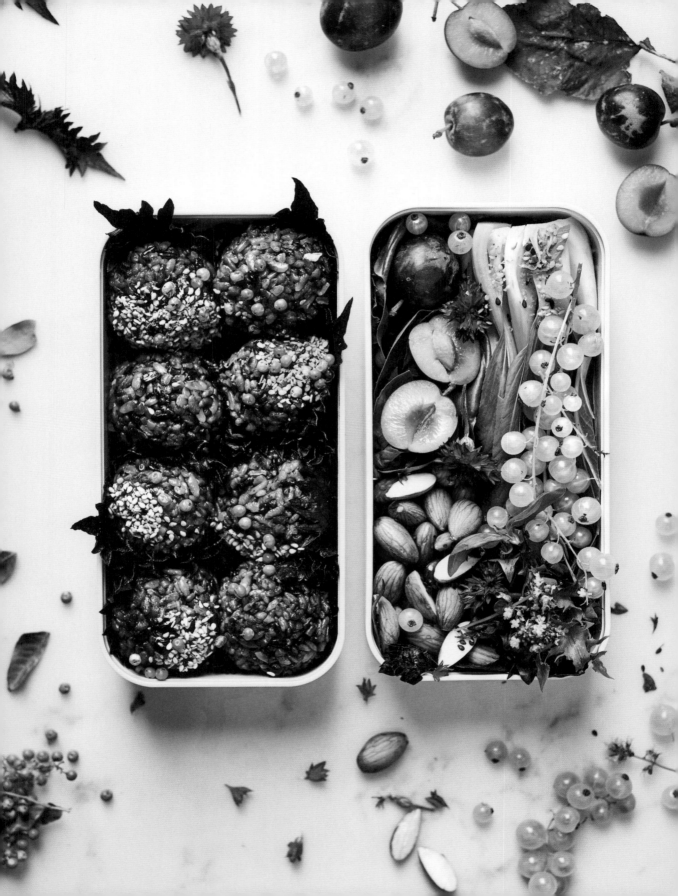

Purple Shiso Mini-onigiri Bento

Since that trip to Japan where I got hold of shiso seeds, I've been growing either green or red shiso every year. Red shiso leaves are tougher than green with a more fruity flavour. Normally they're best cut fine and mixed in to flavour a dish (try with kiwi, lime and brazil nuts in a salad, it's amazing), or dried or preserved, but I think they work really well wrapped around rice balls too! I just had to use purple rice for this bento, contrasted by whitecurrants, which I only get once a year when they're in season at my farmers' market. The pink pepper is a surprise flavouring — its resinous flavour works really well with the red shiso.

Makes 12 mini-onigiri,
2–3 portions.
Eat the same day.

TIPS:
Shiso: Instead of red shiso leaves, use whole radicchio leaves, ripped to size, or nori, cut into about 4 x 8cm strips.

Almonds: Soaked overnight, almonds puff up and become very photogenic (and taste creamier, too).

Onigiri

1 batch of black gradient rice (page 34)
4–5 tbsp white gomashio (page 41), or use the same amount toasted sesame seeds, lightly crushed with ½ tsp sea salt
1 tsp pink peppercorns
12 red shiso leaves (see Tip)
flaky sea salt, smoked if possible, to shape the onigiri

Snip off the shiso stem, close to the leaf. Place the gomashio, or sesame seeds, along with the peppercorns on a small plate, and have a small bowl of water and salt ready.

Wet your hands in the bowl and dab some salt on your palms. Grab a heaped tablespoon of rice and gently but firmly hug it into a ball (rather than roll), using rhythmical hugs (page 114). Wrap the ball in a shiso leaf and dip one side of it in sesame seeds and pink peppercorns (looks more interesting on one side rather than the whole ball) and pack into your box. Repeat until you have 12 balls.

Raw Beauty Box

1 pak choi, trimmed and halved lengthways
a small handful of salad greens
2 tbsp whole almonds, soaked overnight in cold water (see Tip)
2 small Victoria plums
3 purple cornflowers
a few sprigs of flowering thyme
2–3 bunches whitecurrants

Finely shred one half of the pak choi across and mix it with the salad greens to make a bed in the raw beauty box. Lay the second pak choi half on top, cut side-up, and arrange the almonds and plums (whole or cut in half like in the image) in separate sections. Finish with the flowers and currants. To arrange ingredients around the box/es, like in the image, picture the line of movement of one particular ingredient (pink pepper for example), inside the box. Continue this line of movement outside of the box, taking care not to make it look too 'placed'. The ingredients are your brush strokes — be bold and natural!

Rainbow Salad Sushi Roll Bento

I love making nori rolls like this! Raw salad vegetables tightly rolled together, dipped in a spicy dressing – the perfect summer food. If you haven't tried making nori rolls before, I find salad rolls easier than rice ones to start with. The green leaves are your 'rice' here, most lettuce works as long as it's quite soft, thin and pliable. You can use any kind of vegetable or fruit to fill as long as its not too soft or wet. Just cut them into thin long slices. It's quite amazing how much salad you can get into one roll!

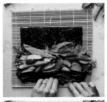
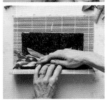
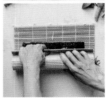
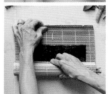
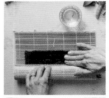
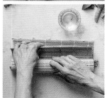
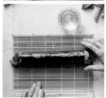

Makes 16 bite-sized pieces, 2 portions.
Fridge life: up to 24 hours.

2 nori sheets
2–6 large salad leaves (enough to cover half a nori sheet in double layers of leaf)
1 each of a small purple, orange and yellow carrot
1 small courgette
a couple of 1–2cm slivers of papaya, or watermelon, deseeded
a few fresh mint or basil leaves
1 avocado, cut into thin slivers
a small handful of green beans, quick-blanched and trimmed, optional

Light dipping sauce:

1 tbsp tamari
juice of ¼ lime
1 hot small chilli (bird's eye), cut in 4 pieces on the diagonal
1 teaspoon maple syrup, optional
a pinch of toasted sesame seeds, any colour (page 41), optional

Creamy dipping sauce:

1 tbsp almond or peanut butter
½ tbsp water
1 tbsp tamari
juice of ¼ lime
1 tsp maple syrup
1cm piece fresh ginger, washed and finely grated

Prepare the fillings

Wash your leaves and pat them dry (very wet leaves will dissolve the nori). Use a julienne slicer, a potato peeler or a sharp knife to slice about half of each carrot into very thin strips lengthways. Do the same with half the courgette. (Store leftover vegetables in an airtight container in the fridge). If you decide to strip the whole of the carrots and courgette, you can use leftovers to make courgetti – toss the strips in dressing, or gomashio and a little lemon and oil.

Fill the roll

It is best to use a sushi mat, but you

can also use a sheet of baking paper, or a clean tea towel laid out on your work surface. Place a nori sheet on top of your mat, shinier side-down. Cover the lower half of the sheet with flattened salad leaves, cut or rip them if needed, to cover as evenly as possible, as this will make it easier to roll. Allow some leaves (and some of the filling) to peek out each end – this will make the finished pieces look pretty.

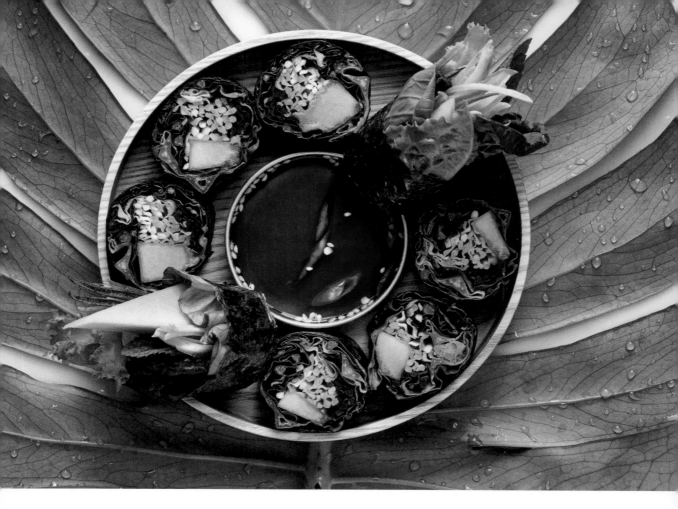

Lay the carrot and courgette strips in an even, horizontal line across the middle of the salad, keeping them as separate as possible colour-wise. Top with strip/s of papaya (or watermelon), mint (or basil) leaves, avocado and green beans, if using. Make sure everything is put in as even thickness as possible.

Roll the roll

Start from the bottom, the edge closest to you (1). Use the mat to start rolling the fillings up, tucking them in with your other hand (2). Focus on bunching up the inside filling into an even and tightly held long sausage as you roll (3). To tighten it, use one hand to hold the mat (and, if possible the nori too) at the top while you pull the sausage towards

you, compacting it (4), then continue rolling.

Once rolled, keep holding it tight, wet a couple of your fingers then wet the top edge of the nori (5), then roll it shut, while still keeping it as tight as possible (6). Leave it to rest for a few moments, seam side-down, before cutting (7).

To cut, use a wet, sharp knife, and cut using quick sawing movements (to ensure the roll doesn't get squashed). Arrange the rolls in your box cut-side up. Place the end rolls either fringy bit up, or lay them down depending on how much space you have.

To make the dipping sauce

Light sauce:

Pour all the ingredients into a small, leak-proof container with a lid.

Creamy sauce:

Stir the nut butter, water, tamari, lime juice and syrup, if using, together in a small, leak-proof container with a lid until smooth. Squeeze the grated ginger to extract the juice straight into the sauce and combine well.

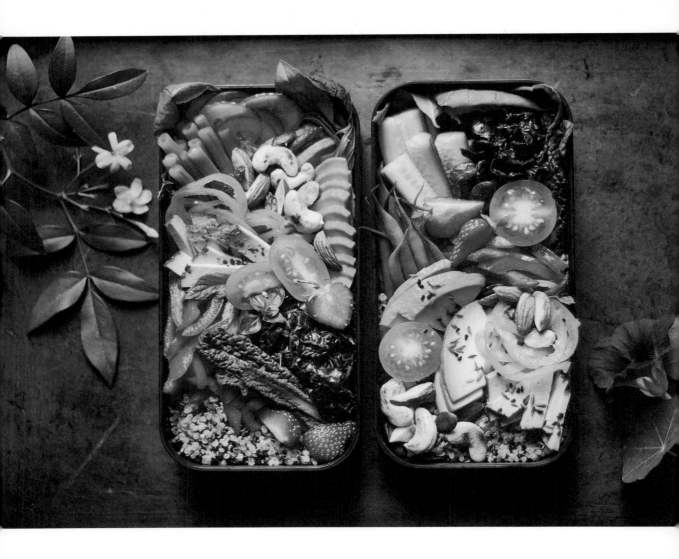

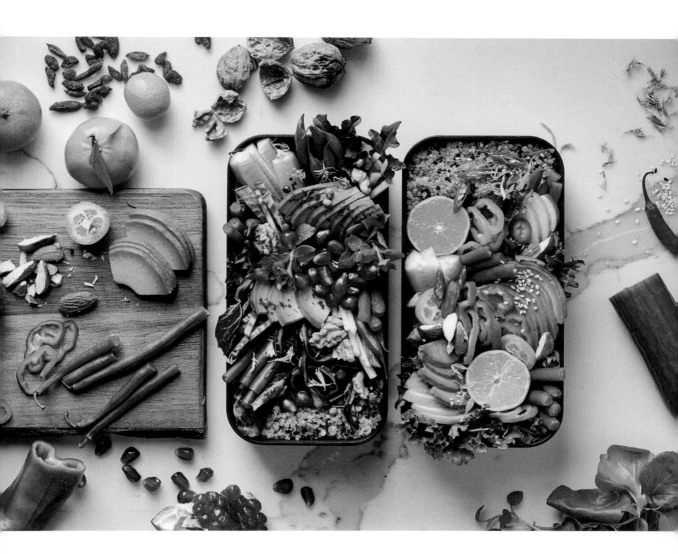

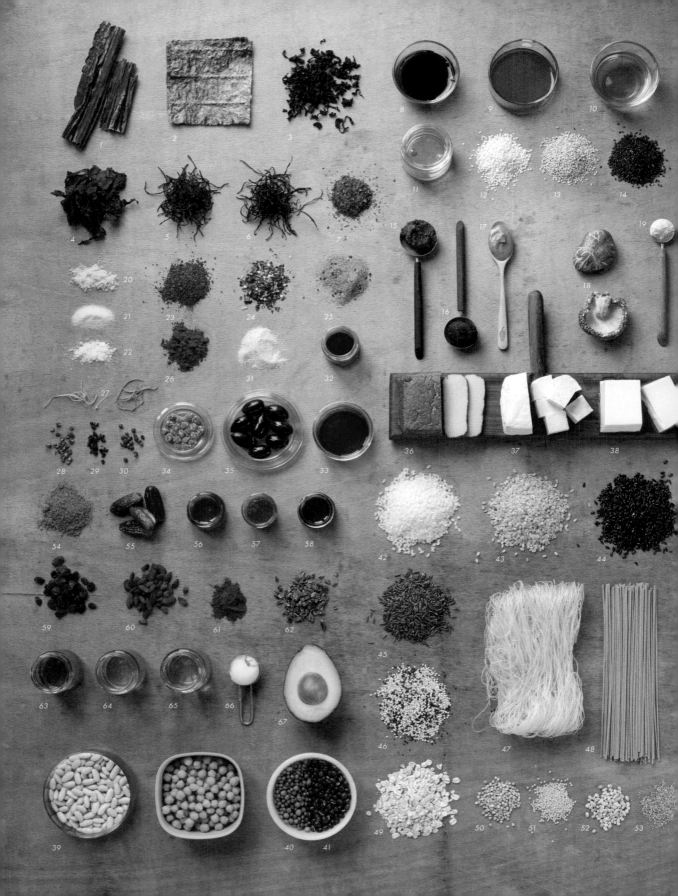

Welcome to my powerful and practical team of helpers that turn simple vegetables into delicious nutritious meals! I have intentionally kept the core ingredients of the recipes of this book to a (fairly) tight group, so, every ingredient can be used in several recipes. When using whole-plant foods as the base of your cooking, the ingredient's quality, including seasonings and condiments, is crucial. Buy the best quality you can afford and enjoy a better powered you, long term! Many of these ingredients can be sourced from supermarkets, others need searching out online or from health-food stores. See Resources on page 191 for the brands I use.

My star helpers are marked*
With these at hand you can make pretty much all of the recipes in this book.

Seaweeds

I often get asked about seaweeds as they may seem quite alien! There's nothing to be scared of though, they are just vegetables from the sea, but powerful ones, charged with umami and mineral powers, soothing properties, and much more. I see them as a combination of a nutritious, natural stock cube and a supercharged veggie that lives in my cupboard (practical!). Buy the best quality you can – a little goes a long way and you want it to be from the cleanest waters possible. Look for deeply, evenly coloured seaweed. My preference is from Japan, Korea or the Atlantic coast. Rather than trying to cut dried seaweed with a knife, use scissors, or chop them up after they've been rehydrated. If you are new to seaweeds, allow your body to get used to them by starting with smaller amounts, then build up as you go.

Kombu* (1)

Kombu is a natural, gentle flavour-enhancer rich in mineral and iodine in particular. Add a 5–10cm piece when cooking grains, pulses, soups and stews. It not only softens pulses' skin but reduces 'gas' too! Typically kombu is removed and often thrown away (!) after it's infused a dish, but I keep mine in to maximise its powers. Look for thick, unbroken kombu with a deep colour.

Nori* (2)

Most know nori as the thin wrap around sushi rolls, but you can roll pretty much anything (that's not too wet) into this edible envelope! High-end nori is thick and a shiny deep green or black with a mellow, complex flavour. Cheaper nori is brown-green, thin and more fishy-tasting, but will still work. Nori sheets normally come in packs of 5–10 (a little crazy considering the amount of packaging used), so I buy mine online in packs of 50, which is a lot cheaper and you'll have more to experiment with. Keep an opened pack in a large ziplock bag, or simply tape it up, as moisture makes nori sad fast. Refresh it by toasting a sheet very briefly over a gas flame.

Wakame* (3)

Wakame is a great place to start if you're new to seaweeds, with its gentle, friendly flavour. I use 'instant' dried wakame (3) in the recipes in this book, which you may recognise from miso soups in Japanese restaurants. It has a lovely, almost emerald green hue when hydrated and is often used generously, almost like salad from the sea! If using non-instant wakame, cut the seaweed strands with scissors before hydrating, and soak for at least double the time stated in the recipe.

Dulse (4)

Deep purple and pretty, dulse adds flavour where fish condiments are normally used – miso soup and Thai dishes, for example (with a 'seawater snowflake' flavour if eaten as is!). It's highly nutritious and often comes wild-harvested. I put it in everything from gomashio (sesame salt) to smoothies! Look for a dark-coloured, slightly moist-looking kind. I prefer whole strands rather than granules.

Hijiki (5) and Arame (6)

Both these are staples in Japanese cusine, but still pretty unknown here in the UK. They're often used as you would a vegetable in cooking (fried, marinated), and have striking long black strands that absorb flavour well. I like adding them dry at the start of cooking grains, too. Hijiki has a slight liquorice flavour and strands a little like soft twigs. Arame has a milder flavour. In my cooking they're interchangeable. They may need crumbling before rehydrating as their strands may be too long to eat. To rehydrate, cover in plenty of cold water in a small bowl for 15–20 minutes.

Aonori (Nori powder) (7)

A humble game changer! A little like a dried parsley of the sea, aonori needs no rehydration, just sprinkle the bright green flakes straight over rice, eggs and tofu, or add it to omelettes or marinades for a touch of sea flavour. Aonori is made from the same seaweed as nori sheets, but processed differently (with a different flavour and colour as a result).

Japanese seasonings

Most of the Japanese seasonings/ condiments I use are fermented (including soy sauce) and bring umami to food as well as microbal goodness. To make the most out of them, don't heat them (if you do, you'll still get their flavour but lose out on some goodness). When using soy-based foods, make sure

you buy them organically produced.

*Soy sauce: Tamari (8) and Shoyu

We all know soy sauce! But there are differences between them. In this book I use tamari, a Japanese soy sauce made without the addition of wheat, making it denser and darker than shoyu (what you'd normally get served in a sushi restaurant) and gluten-free friendly. Despite being less fashionable than tamari right now, I like using shoyu as well, as it has a brighter, little more complex flavour and is cheaper. If you use shoyu instead of tamari in the recipes, use a little more (1 tbsp tamari = 1.5 tbsp shoyu).

Umesu aka Umeshiso, salted plum seasoning (9)

My 'soy sauce' number two! A versatile pink-red liquid salt, clean-tasting, a little fruity and acidic, umesu is the excess liquid from umeboshi pickles – a Japanese national dish. It enhances rather than adds flavour and doesn't colour – which is one reason why I sometimes prefer it to soy sauce. Quick-pickling and marinating is a breeze with umesu – just slice veggies and put them in your bento box, shake a few drops over – and by lunchtime it will have marinated the veggies slightly.

*(Brown) Rice vinegar (10)

My go-to vinegar for quick-pickling, marinades and dressings, rice vinegar is a reliable, mellow team player that doesn't over-power. Choose brown rice vinegar if you can, for a rounder flavour and balance (white rice vinegar can feel a little clinical). If you use apple cider vinegar in the recipes instead, use a little less, 1 tbsp brown rice vinegar = $^2/_3$ tbsp apple cider vinegar.

*Sesame seeds and Toasted sesame oil (11)

Toasted, sesame must be one of the most flavourful seeds there is, and they're highly nutritious too – mineral-rich with a decent protein count. Sesame seeds come in white, hulled (12), whole, unhulled (13) and black (14). Unhulled sesame can be a little bitter, so I tend to alternate between them and white. Black sesame is not so well-known in the UK but it's a staple in Japan, and has a dryer and smokier flavour compared to white – well worth sourcing! I use toasted sesame oil as a flavouring rather than cooking oil (commonly done in Japan too). It is one of those 'magic ingredients' which brings instant deliciousness to anything.

*Miso paste

Not just for soup! Miso is a fermented soy bean paste (mixed with other grains for variety), with a grounding, rounding effect on other flavours, great for everything from filling onigiri rice balls to bringing out the sweetness in treats. Being fermented over long periods (years sometimes), miso teems with friendly microbal life and shouldn't be heated for long. It's perfect for raw foods or for adding to already cooked foods. Miso's colour usually indicates flavour intensity, ranging from very dark and rich (16) to white and sweet (17). In this book I've used brown rice miso (15), a beautiful, medium colour and flavour. If the miso you use is darker or lighter, use a little less, or more in the recipes.

Dried Shiitake mushrooms (18)

I use dried shiitake in a similar way to seaweed, as an all-round flavour enhancer with a subtle Asian-type umami. I tend not to pre-soak, but add them as they are at the start of cooking grains (or soups) and, once they've cooked, I thinly slice them and return them to the food. The stem is very tough, so break it off the dried mushroom and discard before using.

Wasabi powder (19)

Wasabi is well known to all who love sushi and it makes a lovely addition to dressings and marinades too! Mix the powder into a paste and leave for a few minutes before adding to other ingredients (page 49).

Hot, spicy, umami

Since I don't use a lot of garlic or onions, I rely on other ingredients to get that umph. Along with the Japanese condiments listed above, here are my favourites, used throughout the book.

Salt*

I'm a bit of a salt freak! I use fine Guérande sea salt (20), but any sea or rock salt is fine, as long as it has zero additives (eg anti-caking agents) and has had the least amount of natural minerals taken away by processing. Flaky sea salt (22) is processed, but I make an exception as I love its crunchiness as a finishing salt. Each natural salt has a different intensity, and of course every person their own saltiness preference, so use my recipes as a guide. Pictured is also Pink Himalayan salt (21).

Gochugaru* (Korean pepper) (23)

Gochugaru is always an instant hit at my workshops! I can't remember when I first started using it but I've been buying it in 500g bags ever since... It is most famously known as the red pepper powder used in kimchi, Korean fermented cabbage. It's mild-hot with a unique round sweetness and I warmly recommend trying to source it. A substitute blend is listed in the recipes or just use chilli flakes, but use less.

Chilli flakes* (24)

Chilli flakes, aka crushed red pepper, are my go-to chilli (when not using gochugaru). They have a clean, easy to distribute heat which goes well with other flavours.

Shichimi Tōgarashi (25)

A Japanese 7-spice mix with a unique, citrussy heat – great as a pretty finishing touch or sprinkled on soba noodles.

Spanish smoked paprika (26)

This has a gorgeous smoky flavour and warm colour. It is great mixed with other seasonings, including soy sauce and miso.

Citrus peel (27)

I love adding a scrape of citrus to food, which adds brightness without acidity. I buy organic (but often get 'normal' for juice). If you can't get organic (even if it is unwaxed), scrub the skin throughly with a drop of washing-up liquid to remove potential pesticides before using. A small handheld citrus zester is very handy, but you can also use a fine box grater.

Sanshō pepper and Sichuan pepper

Citrussy and uniquely tongue-tingling, Japanese Sanshō (28) is interchangeable with the easier-to-source Chinese Sichuan (29). Only a few crushed peppercorns are needed (test before using as very fresh corns can be overpowering!) and are best used with neutral flavours like rice, noodles or greens (I've used them in mixed blessings onigiri on page 112).

Pink peppercorns (30)

They bring pretty colour and little bursts of resinous flavour as a finishing touch to a bento. They shine, used in moderation.

Garlic granules (31)

Even a small pinch of these small specks of dried garlic add a rounded, warming umami to food. They are less overpowering than raw.

Liquid smoke (32)

Easier to source than you may think and a gamechanger in the kitchen! Liquid smoke is made by simply collecting the residue from natural, burning wood and makes your food taste like bacon (or better actually!). It adds a drying, 'grilled' element to bento.

Fish sauce (vegetarian) (33)

I recently discovered this alternative, based on soy beans. The original, fish version is essential in South-East Asian cooking for an intensely savoury flavour that complements spicy and sour foods. When used as a marinade for tofu and mushrooms it brings out a really 'meaty' element!

Capers (34) and Olives (35)

Anything that's small and savoury, naturally preserved and can be used right away is great for bento. Both these are available to buy in glass rather than plastic = extra earth points!

Tofu

A love-hate object of healthy eating... claimed to be everything from bland to adversely affecting hormonal balance. To me, organic tofu is a practical and versatile food when eaten in moderation, especially as I'm not relying on animal products. I use it in a bunch of recipes here – hopefully those should help with the 'bland' issue!

Firm, smoked Tofu* (36)

If you find tofu wobbly and meh, you must try it smoked! The texture and flavour is similar to some processed meats (sorry), it's concentrated (you only need a little) and it doesn't spoil as quickly as softer tofu – so it's great to have on hand for bento. Keep an opened pack in an airtight container and it will last even longer.

Soft-medium Tofu (37)

This is the type you'll find when you buy 'regular' tofu (and may be the one which has given tofu some of it's bad rep – it needs a little help to shine!). Try freezing it first (see page 150) or marinating then frying or roasting. When done right, it's lovely.

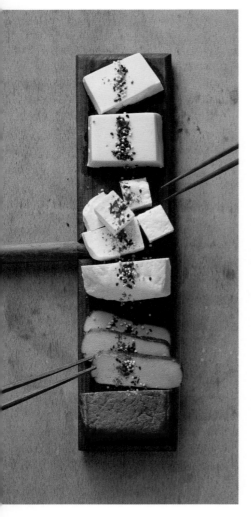

Silken Tofu (38)

Silken tofu in tetrapak keeps for months – great 'emergency food'! It can be eaten without cooking first, but needs generous seasoning, like in the hiya-yakko bento (page 78).

Beans + how to cook

Canned beans are handy (and I use them a lot), but when you cook your own it's a whole new level of tasty – almost a different food! (39) It was rare that I did though, until I found out you can *freeze* beans once cooked. It now makes sense to go through the relative faff that is cooking beans to have tasty, inexpensive (and less waste!) beans at hand. To improve digestibility (and reduce the amount of gas pulses produce) this is my process:

1. Soak. I make large batches of beans, starting with 500–1kg dry beans. Soak in cold water for 10–12 hours. During this time, change the water to fresh as many times as possible (at least 2–3 times), as some of the 'fart particles' will seep into the water.

2. Two-step cooking. Start with fresh water, boil the beans hard for 15–20 minutes without a lid (to allow some of those fart particles to evaporate into the air), then discard the cooking water (I think you know why by now). Add fresh water and a 10–15cm piece of kombu (which softens the beans' skin and improves digestibility) and simmer, covered, until the beans are soft but not mushy. I let the beans cool in the water (contradictory, I know, but I find this makes a moister, tastier bean). The kombu can be finely chopped and added back into the beans for extra nutrients.

3. Freeze. Once cool, rinse the beans clean in a strainer under the tap then pack in plastic (reused) bags. I tend to pack roughly the same volume as a

can of beans. Flatten your bean-bags before closing (this makes them defrost quicker), then freeze. They will last a couple of months before they start to lose their flavour.

4. Defrost. Either defrost overnight in the fridge or quick-defrost by immersing the closed bag in cold water. If you are using the beans for a hot meal, you can add them frozen to the cooking food.

Mung beans (40) and Aduki beans (41)

Both these varieties are small and cook quite fast, so I like using them in some of the mixed-grain rice or one-pot rice recipes (pages 32–37). Mung beans are also one of the easiest beans to sprout (whereas aduki is one of the hardest!), like in the zen bento (page 136).

Rice, grains and noodles

White Japanese rice* (Sushi rice) (42)

It's called sushi rice in the UK, but when it's not made with sushi seasoning it's really just 'Japanese rice'. What's available in the UK isn't actually grown in Japan (and if it is, it's a very premium price), but Italy grows a lot of good-quality 'Japonica' and I recommend buying that, rather than U.S.- or Chinese- produced rice where the growing regulations are less strict than in the EU. You save on air miles, too! I buy 10kg bags online to save on both packaging and price. As a cash-strapped student I'd sometimes buy inexpensive pudding rice, which, if washed and cooked like white Japanese rice, comes out quite well.

Brown Short Grain Rice* (43)

I was first introduced to brown short-grain rice whilst working in a London health-food shop. Having come from living in Japan, this rice was very similar to the (rare) brown rice there. Just like white, it is often grown in Italy and mostly produced organically, so it's a great staple.

Black Rice (44)

I love mixing black rice with my white or brown (pages 28–30). In this book, 'black rice' refers to Italian Venus rice, also called Nerone or Verene. It is wholegrain, so adds fibre and minerals as well as gorgeous purply colour.

Red rice (45)

Another gorgeous-coloured wholegrain rice, which comes in a few varieties. Camargue and red Thai are the ones I've used so far – lovely on their own or mixed in with white or brown rice.

Quinoa* (46)

A classic 'health food' and for a good reason! It's high in protein and, if cooked right, delicious too. Quinoa tastes good even after being refrigerated (whilst rice gets hard and dry and needs heating up), making it a great bento-staple.

Dry rice vermicelli* (47)

I always keep a packet in my cupboard for when I have no grains prepared, or when I want to whip up a big cold noodle salad. They take minutes to rehydrate and generally don't stick together when cold, making them great for bento. Rehydrated, they keep up to 5 days in an airtight container in the fridge –and they are easy to dress or added to soups or stir-fry. I prefer the ones produced in Thailand or Vietnam. Check the ingredients list and get the ones made from just, 'rice, water'.

Soba noodles (48)

A Japanese classic, soba are made from a mix of buckwheat and wheat flour, which makes them a warm grey colour with a delicious bite. The 100% buckwheat soba are gluten-free, stickier

and more fragile when cooked.

Rolled Oats

We go through crazy amounts of oats at home. They're nutritionally balanced and I find them very gentle and friendly for digestion too. Oats are made into flakes by steam-rolling and I prefer 'Jumbo Oats' (49) as they are rolled the thickest, making them oxidise slower (compared to porridge oats or instant oats) as they stay closer to their original, natural shape.

Buckwheat (50)

Cute, triangular shaped and gluten-free, these are great mixed in with white or brown rice, adding a moist, slightly 'slidy' character and nutrients. Toasted, it adds great crunch, like in savoury granola (page 43). I find buckwheat best mixed with other ingredients.

Millet (51)

It is a yellow-coloured, small round grain, high in protein and iron with a satisfying crunch when toasted. I use it sparingly mixed in with other grains.

Pearl barley (52) and Amaranth (53)

Both are delicious cooked with other grains. Pearl barley (not gluten free) adds small chewy, puffy pillows to your rice and a handful of amaranth makes your rice sticky with their tiny, round grains (very cute), whilst adding lots of valuable nutrients.

Natural sweeteners

I feel strongly about teaching one's body to accept and thrive on lower levels of sweetness than what is 'normal' in our food culture right now. When my relationship to food was very imbalanced I found that intense sweetness triggered binge-eating and terrible mood and energy swings.

Gradually, I've weaned myself off (with many fails along the way) and these days I simply don't enjoy overly sweet foods. Partly because I know how strong of an effect it will have on me (short-lived high, exhaustion, feeling empty/lacking). But I still enjoy sweetness. I'm just careful which sweeteners, and what amounts, keep me balanced. Here are my staples.

To substitute sweeteners in my recipes: 1 tsp coconut sugar = 1 tsp rice malt syrup = ½ tsp clear honey = ½ tsp maple syrup = ½ tsp agave syrup = ½ tsp regular sugar.

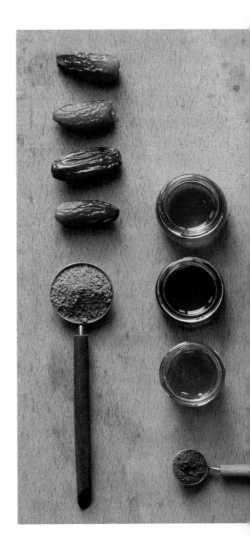

Coconut palm sugar* (54)

My go-to sugar, for many reasons. It is not overly sweet, has a rounded caramelly flavour and is very easy to cook with (even added to savoury foods). It is made from the sap of coconut palm blossoms (much like maple syrup), simply boiled down into crystals. Nothing is taken out apart from moisture, meaning you get the rest of the goodness from the sap, too! It is considered a sustainable sugar, as the palms are not damaged in the process, and the sugar needs to be made on site (near the palms), meaning the palm-farmers get paid better for their crop. Finally, out of all the 'natural sugars' out there, it is one of the most affordable ones! Win × many!

Dates

I rarely eat dates on their own, but I use them to sweeten foods a lot! Being a whole fruit, their sugar is embedded in fibre, complex carbs and more, meaning they release more slowly into your bloodstream compared to pure (refined) sugar. Plus, you get all the other nutrients a date contains! Whole dates may seem less convenient than other sweeteners, but if you view them as a concentrated sweetening and thickening ingredient then it's easy to know how to use them. In my recipes I use deglet nour (55), which are half the size, less sweet and less expensive than Medjool. Whenever I can, I give my dates (and any dry fruit) a wash before adding them to foods. Their journey to your kitchen has been a long one!

Honey (56)

My true love. Bees naturally produce an excess of honey and good beekeepers (who I respect a lot) will leave enough for the bees to thrive, and make sure they are healthy while they do their very important job of pollinating plants, fruits and crops. I buy honey that's either organic (there are many more regulations around how bees can be kept and treated when organic) or produced by small, independent bee-keepers, including local London honey!

Brown rice syrup (57)

I never 'got' this brown sweetener until I discovered that their subtle, malty flavour and viscousness take treats to the next level, like in the matcha brownies (page 68). Use like-for-like as coconut palm sugar in recipes.

Maple syrup

Maple syrup (58) is a lovely treat sweetener to me, or one to use when a recipe needs a thin-flowing syrup.

Agave syrup

I use agave when I want to keep a light colour in a dish. In my recipes you can substitute maple with agave like-for-like.

Sultanas and Goji berries

Sultanas are my affordable, dried fruit I use to sweeten nut mixes and breakfasts, and goji berries are my fancy ones. I love how this ingredient instantly adds a missing red element to a bento.

Vanilla

A pinch of vanilla is often all it takes to connect all the flavours togther in a sweet dish. I use ground-up whole vanilla pods, sold as a moist powder, where nothing has been wasted.

Oils

Olive oil * (63)

A classic. I use extra virgin olive oil, the best, organic quality I can afford.

Flaxseed oil (64)

This has been a loyal companion for years. Flaxseed oil is rich in the omegas you'd normally get from oily fish. Good flaxseed oil smells and tastes fresh (not bitter). I've found it has a positive effect on my skin and on feeling hydrated in general. I crave it when I haven't had it for a while! Use it unheated, as you would extra virgin olive oil – in salads, on rice with salt or on bread.

Toasted sesame oil – see Japanese condiments

'A little oil, to fry' (65)

I alternate between extra virgin olive oil and organic grapeseed oil. Grapeseed oil has the higher smoke point.

Avocado (67)

Much of the food in my bento is prepared without oils, so I like using avocado as a fat element. It binds salad veggies together, often with seasoned crunchy nuts and seeds. Try to buy avocados that are grown as locally to you as possible.

Eggs

For all my vegan friends, I've chosen to include all the recipes that represent the past years of making bento for Andy and lunches for myself. In those, organic eggs have often featured and been much loved! They are the one animal-based food I still don't feel (too) strange eating. The eggs we buy are all organic, most of the time from our farmers' market. There's a huge difference between those and 'normal', battery farmed eggs, both in the way they've been produced and how they taste. Still, it's not an ideal situation to mistreat other creatures en masse just so we can fill our bellies in a way we're accustomed to. For the moment, the very least I can do is to support smaller-scale, gentler-produced organic producers!

Fresh Potions

Edible Flowers and Leaves

Being on Instagram opened my eyes (quite literally) to edible flowers and I love how they bring magic to anything they're added to. In winter, I like dried cornflower petals for a pop of colour. In the image on the right you can see some of the goodies I've grown (or found wild) in our garden:
Thyme flowers, dill flowers, wood sorrel leaves (wild), purple and pink corn flowers, nasturitums, rocket flowers, pansies, lavender flowers, forget-me-nots (wild) and mustard green flowers.

Pomegranate

While in season, I'll always have a pomegranate on the go in my fridge (my winter berries!) as they add instant red sparkle with little bursts of zesty juice, packed with antioxidants too. Gently score a section of the skin of a pomegranate to tear some off (and with it, a bunch of seed segments), then pick as many as needed and keep the rest in a bowl in the fridge. This way, one fruit can last for weeks. They're sold without any packaging, which makes me love them even more.

Summer Berries

Growing up in the north of Sweden, no fruit trees would survive, but hardy little shrubs made up for it with masses of berries! They have a special place in my heart still, and in summer, they're great for bento. Sadly packaging is an issue with fresh berries (lots of packaging, short enjoyment) so they're only an occasional treat.

Leaf Spa

Give your leaves some love in a Leaf Spa! Many of my recipes say 'a handful of salad leaves' and if you prepare them like this, restaurant prep-style, they get crunchier, longer lasting and are just a grab away from your bento box. Use a base of sturdier (and more inexpensive) salad heads and add accents of herbs or coloured leaves. Baby spinach or rocket from the supermarket go soggy fast so are better avoided in the spa.

Fridge life up to 1 week.

Lettuce, cut or torn into bite-sized pieces
Kale, torn into bite-sized chunks
Pak choi or tatsoi cut into bite-sized pieces
Sturdier herbs like parsley, mint, dill, torn into bite-sized pieces
Radicchio, torn into bite-sized chunks
Chicory, whole leaves stripped off
The leafy part of celery, beetroot or fennel

Wash your leaves and use a salad spinner to dry them. Place a damp paper towel in the base of a big plastic box, and either tear the leaves straight in, or first cut then transfer. Cover with another damp paper towel, close the lid and store in the fridge.

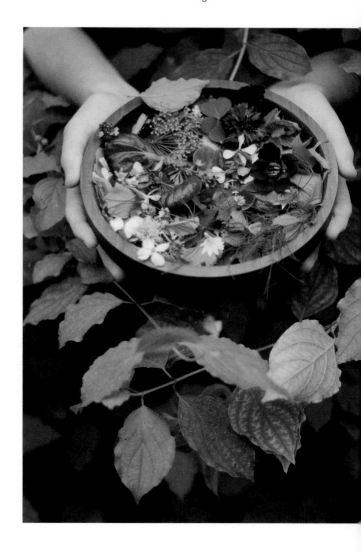

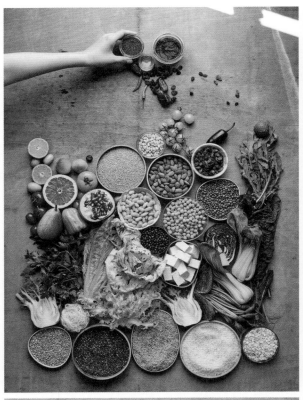

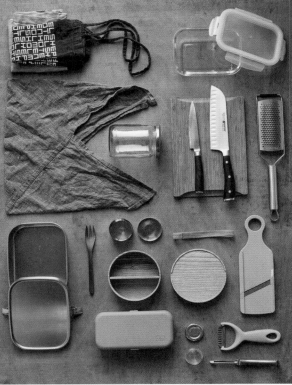

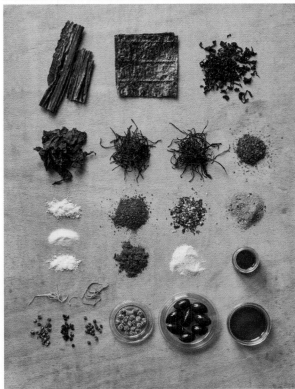

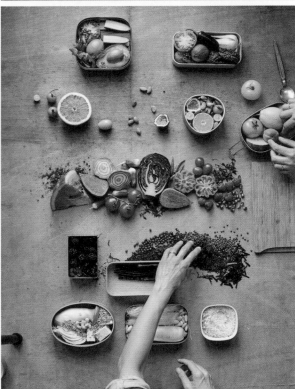

RESOURCES

Bento boxes and food storage

Bamboo round bento box: *Swiss Advance*
Enamel storage containers, also used as bento boxes: *Noda Horo* (Japan import)
Glass storage containers, also used as bento boxes: *Lock & Lock*
Plastic bento boxes (pictured left): *Monbento*
Stainless steel bento boxes, small stainless steel containers for snacks: *UKonserve*
Stainless steel bento boxes, silicon seal (pictured left): *Aizawa* (Japan import)
Stainless steel bento boxes, steel lid: *A Slice of Green*
Wax wraps: *Abeego Beewax Food Wraps*
Wooden (Ash) round bento boxes (pictured left): *Eshly Deli Box*
Wooden (bent cedar) oval bento box: *Search 'mage wappa' or 'wappa bento'*
All my other bento boxes are Japanese made, and bought in Japan.

Furoshiki, bento bags, linen

Furoshiki used in images: *Link Collective*, artisan made in Japan
Furoshiki used in images (sold as large linen napkin, pictured left) plus aprons and clothing: *Not Perfect Linen*, Etsy
Bento bags: *Sorabento*, Etsy (pictured left)
Large furoshiki, fabric produce shopping bags, aprons: *The Organic Company*

Kitchen tools and kitchen ware

Bamboo chopping board (pictured left), fork and spoon: *Bambu*
Bamboo eco fibre bowls: *Ekobo*
Blender with herb attachment: *Magimix*
Brass/wood measuring spoons: *Facturegoods*
Citrus zester: *Brabantia*
Coconut wood forks: *Coconut Bowls*
Enamel mixing bowls: *Falcon*, their simple 'catering' lines
Grater, hand held (pictured): *Microplane*
Japanese vegetable/scrubbing brush *search: Tawashi brush*
Julienne peeler (pictured left): *Kiwi Pro Slice*, Thai Papaya Slicer
Knife (pictured left): *Wüsthof* 'Classic Icon' and *Richardson Sheffield* 'Midori'
Mandolin (pictured left) and julienner: *Ai Kyogo*, Q series (Japan import)
Salad spinner: 'Herb spinner', *OXO*
Twig spoons: Pamela Schroeder, *Aboda*

Clothing and accessories

Jewellery worn in the images: *Marcia Vidal Jewellery*, made in London
Pink dress and yellow top worn in the images: *LF Markey*, designed in London

Places to shop

British grown and organic: *Growing Communities Farmers' Market* (every Saturday), Stoke Newington, London
Staples in bulk *buywholefoodsonline.com*
Sustainable food prep and storage *asliceofgreen.co.uk*
Japanese seasonings (including tamari, miso, umesu, brown rice vinegar, toasted sesame oil), brown rice syrup, dry shiitake, seaweeds, silken tofu: *clearspring.co.uk* (their products were mostly used when creating these recipes)
Japanese kitchen tools: *Kitchen Provisions*

Foodstuffs

Many of the brands listed here are available at supermarkets, in health food shop and online.
Black Venus rice: *Biona*
Bulk whole foods, including specialist foods: grains (including brown short grain rice, puffed quinoa), seeds (including sesame), salts and much more *Buywholefoodsonline.com*
Cashews, almonds in 500g bags: *supermarkets'* own Asian/Indian brands
Chipotle chilli: *Cool Chile Company*
Dry rice vermicelli: most *supermarkets*
Dulse: *Emerald Isle Seaweed*
Fish sauce (vegetarian): *24Vegan.com*
Flax oil: *Biona*
Gochugaru: *Tae Kyung* brand
Liquid smoke: *The Original Australian*
Mushrooms, unusual: *Smithy Mushrooms*
Nori: *search: 50 Sheets, Korean made*
Sanshō pepper: *Spice Mountain*
Sauerkraut: *Pama Creations*
Shichimi Tōgarashi: at *Japan Centre*
Sichuan pepper: *Steenbergs*
Smoked, firm tofu: *Taifun or Viana*
Soft-medium tofu: *Clearspot, Cauldron*
Spanish smoked paprika: all *supermarkets*
Specialist foods: Wholefoods, London
Vanilla: *Ndali*, whole bean powder
Wakame, instant: *Wel-Pac*
White Japanese rice: *Haruka*, 10kg (Italy)

ACKNOWLEDGEMENTS

Thank you,

Andy, for being the best life partner I could wish for. Meowth, Tigger and little Porridge for being the sweetest, furriest company the many days and nights I spent working on this book. My family, with its many extended arms, for giving me a loving, stimulating start in life and supporting me in so many different ways, up to this day. My whooooole Instagram community – without your support, love and inspiration, Bento Power would never be. Takaya-san for opening their home to my 17-year old self and introducing Japanese family life to me, including bento. My Japanese father and his wife, who, even though our contact is sparse, unknowingly influenced much of my recent 'career change' during our last two visits. My friends and fellow students in Japan of who many I've lost contact with, but who live on in my understanding of the world. Kyle Books for believing in Bento Power and giving me the opportunity to create this book, for your knowledge and patience and the creative freedom you've entrusted me with. My literary agent Jonathan Conway for understanding me and my ideas so well and Ben(to) Lethbridge for connecting us. Nicki of Before Breakfast Design for being my dream designer. Niki Webster and Lisa Dawson for joining me at a crazed moment of recipe-testing and starting to shoot, and Amélie Marquis-Angulo for helping me realise some of the photography I'm the most happy with in this book. Carolina Llamusi-Silbermann for being able to catch me looking natural in portraits and Jenna Foxton for giving me some cool. Bettina Campolucci-Bordi for leading the way in becoming a 'full-time foodie', and all my other insta-sisters and brothers who have given me some of themselves, which can be seen on the pages of this book. Mayuka Hulmes for being my personal Tokyo bento-box shopper, and everyone else who have given generously of their time, expertise, gifts and support to bring Bento Power into the world!

All opinions and interpretations of Japanese culture and customs are my own, based on living and studying there for 3.5 years. If I got something wrong, I'm sorry! I'd also like to express huge gratitude and respect to the other food cultures I've had the pleasure to be influenced by including Korean, South-east Asian, Bulgarian and Swedish.

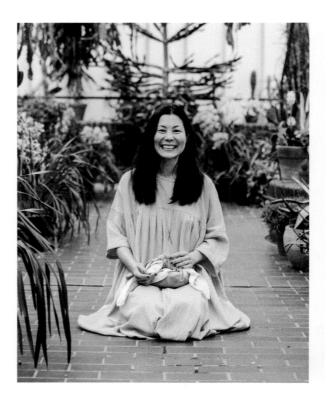

Sara Kiyo Popowa

of

Shiso Delicious

Sara is a photographer and recipe developer based in London, known for her colourful, plant-celebrating bento lunch boxes on Instagram. She created Shiso Delicious to inspire beauty, sustainability and appreciation on every level in life through food and lifestyle.

www.shisodelicious.com
@shisodelicious
@bentoparty

#bentopowerbook